Pat Precin, MS, OTR/L
Editor

Healing 9/11:
Creative Programming
by Occupational Therapists

Healing 9/11: Creative Programming by Occupational Therapists has been co-published simultaneously as *Occupational Therapy in Mental Health*, Volume 21, Numbers 3/4 2006.

Pre-publication
REVIEWS,
COMMENTARIES,
EVALUATIONS . . .

"**G**IVES READERS VALUABLE IN-
SIGHTS into the crucial work
of skilled helpers–with children, firefighters, psychiatric patients, displaced
workers, burn victims, and more–
true stories of people helping people cope with and transcend the pain
of September 11."

Scott Bennett, MSEd, MSW
Author of The Elements of Résumé
Style

The Haworth Press, Inc.

Healing 9/11:
Creative Programming
by Occupational Therapists

Healing 9/11: Creative Programming by Occupational Therapists has been co-published simultaneously as *Occupational Therapy in Mental Health*, Volume 21, Numbers 3/4 2006.

Healing 9/11: Creative Programming by Occupational Therapists, edited by Pat Precin, MS, OTR/L (Vol. 21, No. 3/4, 2006). *"GIVES READERS VALUABLE INSIGHTS into the crucial work of skilled helpers–with children, firefighters, psychiatric patients, displaced workers, burn victims, and more–true stories of people helping people cope with and transcend the pain of September 11." (Scott Bennett, MSEd, MSW, Author of* The Elements of Résumé Style)

Occupational Therapy in Forensic Psychiatry: Role Development and Schizophrenia, by Victoria P. Schindler, PhD, OTR (Vol. 20, No. 3/4, 2004). *"DR. SCHINDLER HAS ANSWERED OUR PROFESSION'S CALL for more evidence-based practice by using both basic and applied scientific inquiry to investigate how individuals diagnosed with schizophrenia can develop meaningful life roles while in a maximum-security psychiatric facility. Her findings clearly demonstrate the value of focusing intervention on helping clients pursue meaningful occupations through role development, rather than simply focusing on individual components of treatment." (Laurie Knis-Matthews, OT, MA, Assistant Professor, Kean University)*

Surviving 9/11: Impact and Experiences of Occupational Therapy Practitioners, edited by Pat Precin, MS, OTR/L (Vol. 19, No. 3/4, 2003). *Analyzes the many roles occupational therapy practitioners played during the tragic events of 9/11; examines new therapeutic practices developed because of the terrorist attacks.*

An Ethnographic Study of Mental Health Treatment and Outcomes: Doing What Works, by Fran Babiss, PhD, OTR/L (Vol. 18, No. 3/4, 2002). *"All mental health clinicians and scholars will find this book INSIGHTFUL AND PROVOCATIVE. This book contains more than a description of three women living with anorexia nervosa; the rich qualitative data captures their pain and their struggles with daily life to survive." (Jim Hinojosa, PhD, OT, FAOTA, Professor and Chair, Department of Occupational Therapy, New York University)*

Recovery and Wellness: Models of Hope and Empowerment for People with Mental Illness, edited by Catana Brown, PhD, OTR/L, FAOTA (Vol. 17, No. 3/4, 2001). *Provides guidelines for incorporating wellness and recovery principles into mental health services using the Recovery Model.*

Domestic Abuse Across the Lifespan: The Role of Occupational Therapy, by Christine A. Helfrich, PhD, OTR/L (Vol. 16, No. 3/4, 2001). *"For those occupational therapists who view themselves as holistic service providers, this book is a must-read. . . . Includes examples, studies, and research results." (Linda T. Learneard, OTR/L, President, Occupational Therapy Consultation and Rehabilitation Services, Inc.)*

Brain Injury and Gender Role Strain: Rebuilding Adult Lifestyles After Injury, by Sharon A. Gutman, PhD, OTR (Vol. 15, No. 3/4, 2000). *"Dr. Gutman has developed an innovative target setting and treatment planning protocol that focuses the therapist on the key areas of concern. I highly recommend this book to therapists who work with clients in the post-acute period of recovery from TBI." (Gordon Muir Giles, MA, Dip COT, OTR, Director of Neurobehavioral Services, Crestwood Behavioral Health, Inc., and Assistant Professor, Samuel Merritt College, Oakland, California)*

New Frontiers in Psychosocial Occupational Therapy, edited by Anne Hiller Scott, PhD, OTR, FAOTA (Vol. 14, No. 1/2, 1998). *"Speaks a clear message about mental health practice in occupational therapy, shattering old visions of practice to insights about empowerment and advocacy." (Sharan L. Schwartzberg, EdD, OTR, FAOTA, Professor and Chair, Boston School of Occupational Therapy, Tufts University)*

Evaluation and Treatment of the Psychogeriatric Patient, edited by Diane Gibson, MS, OTR (Vol. 10, No. 3, 1991). *"Occupational therapists everywhere, learners and sophisticates alike, and in-hospital and out-patient areas as well as home-bound and home-active, would enjoy and profit from this exposition as much as I did." (American Association of Psychiatric Administrators)*

Student Recruitment in Psychosocial Occupational Therapy: Intergenerational Approaches, edited by Susan Haiman (Vol. 10, No. 1, 1990). *"Can serve to enlighten both academics and clinicians as to their roles in attracting students to become practitioners in mental health settings. Each article could well serve as a catalyst for discussion in the classroom or clinic." (Canadian Journal of Occupational Therapy)*

Group Protocols: A Psychosocial Compendium, edited by Susan Haiman (Vol. 9, No. 4, 1990). *"Presents succinct protocols for a wide range of groups that are typically run by activities therapists, vocational counselors, art therapists, and other mental health professionals." (International Journal of Group Psychotherapy)*

Instrument Development in Occupational Therapy, edited by Janet Hawkins Watts and Chestina Brollier (Vol. 8, No. 4, 1989). *Examines content and concurrent validity and development of the Assessment of Occupational Functioning (AOF), and carefully compares the AOF with a similar instrument, the Occupational Case Analysis Interview and Rating Scale (OCAIRS), to discover the similarities and strengths of these instruments.*

Group Process and Structure in Psychosocial Occupational Therapy, edited by Diane Gibson, MS, OTR (Vol. 8, No. 3, 1989). *Highly skilled professionals examine the important concepts of group therapy to help build cohesive, safe groups.*

Treatment of Substance Abuse: Psychosocial Occupational Therapy Approaches, edited by Diane Gibson, MS, OTR (Vol. 8, No. 2, 1989). *A unique overview of contemporary assessment and rehabilitation of alcohol and chemical dependent substance abusers.*

The Development of Standardized Clinical Evaluations in Mental Health, Principal Investigator: Noomi Katz, PhD, OTR; edited by Claudia Kay Allen, MA, OTR, FAOTA; Commentator: Janice P. Burke, MA, OTR, FAOTA (Vol. 8, No. 1, 1988). *"Contains a collection of research-based articles encompassing several evaluations that can be used by occupational therapists practicing in mental health." (American Journal of Occupational Therapy)*

Evaluation and Treatment of Adolescents and Children, edited by Diane Gibson, MS, OTR (Vol. 7, No. 2, 1987). *Experts share research results and practices that have proven successful in helping young people who suffer from psychiatric and medical disorders.*

Treatment of the Chronic Schizophrenic Patient, edited by Diane Gibson, MS, OTR (Vol. 6, No. 2, 1986). *"Reflect[s] creative and fresh concepts of current treatment for the chronically mentally ill. . . . Recommended for the therapist practicing in psychiatry." (Canadian Journal of Occupational Therapy)*

The Evaluation and Treatment of Eating Disorders, edited by Diane Gibson, MS, OTR (Vol. 6, No. 1, 1986). *"A wealth of information. . . . Covers the subject thoroughly. . . . This book, well-conceived and well-written, is recommended not only for clinicians working with clients with anorexia nervosa and bulimia but for all therapists who wish to become acquainted with the subject of eating disorders in general." (Library Journal)*

Philosophical and Historical Roots of Occupational Therapy, edited by Karen Diasio Serrett (Vol. 5, No. 3, 1985). *"Recommended as an easy-to-get-through background read for occupational therapists and for generalists wishing a fuller acquaintance with the backdrop of occupational therapy." (Rehabilitation Literature)*

Short-Term Treatment in Occupational Therapy, edited by Diane Gibson, MS, OTR, and Kathy Kaplan, MS, OTR (Vol. 4, No. 3, 1984). *"Thought provoking and relevant to various issues facing OTs in a short term inpatient psychiatric setting. . . . Very readable . . . concise, well-written, and stimulating." (Canadian Journal of Occupational Therapy)*

SCORE: Solving Community Obstacles and Restoring Employment, by Lynn Wechsler Kramer, MS, OTR (Vol. 4, No. 1, 1984). *"This needed book is an effective instrument for occupational therapists wanting to 'teach employable handicapped how to obtain a job in a competitive (labor) market.' Very relevant to professional practice . . . a useful how-to instrument." (The American Journal of Occupational Therapy)*

Occupational Therapy with Borderline Patients, edited by Diane Gibson, MS, OTR (Vol. 3, No. 3, 1983). *"Offers clinicians an opportunity to review current theoretical concepts, management, and design of activity groups for this population. Well written . . . provides good reference lists and well-developed discussions." (The American Journal of Occupational Therapy)*

Healing 9/11:
Creative Programming
by Occupational Therapists

Pat Precin, MS, OTR/L
Editor

Healing 9/11: Creative Programming by Occupational Therapists has been co-published simultaneously as *Occupational Therapy in Mental Health*, Volume 21, Numbers 3/4 2006.

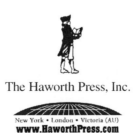

The Haworth Press, Inc.

New York • London • Victoria (AU)
www.HaworthPress.com

Healing 9/11: Creative Programming by Occupational Therapists
has been co-published simultaneously as *Occupational Therapy in
Mental Health*, Volume 21, Numbers 3/4 2006.

Cover design by Kerry Mack.

Cover photo, "Gone, But Not Forgotten," by Fran Babiss.

Library of Congress Cataloging-in-Publication Data

Healing 9/11 : creative programming by occupational therapists / Pat Precin, editor.
     p. cm.
    "Co-published simultaneously as Occupational therapy in mental health, volume 21, numbers
3/4 2006."
    Includes bibliographical references and index.
    ISBN-13: 978-0-7890-2362-9 (hard cover : alk. paper)
    ISBN-13: 978-0-7890-2363-6 (soft cover : alk. paper)
    1. Occupational therapy. 2. Crisis intervention (Mental health services) 3. September 11 Terror-
ist Attacks, 2001–Psychological aspects. 4. Disaster victims–Mental health. I. Precin, Pat. II. Occupational therapy in mental health. III. Title: Healing nine/eleven. [DNLM: 1. September 11 Terrorist
Attacks–psychology–New York City. 2. Occupational Therapy–methods–New York City. 3. Crisis Intervention–methods–New York City. 4. Stress Disorders, Post-Traumatic–psychology–New York
City. 5. Stress Disorders, Post-Traumatic–therapy–New York City. W1 OC601N v.21 no.3/4 2006 /
WM 170 H4344 2006]

RM735.H355 2006
362.2'04251–dc22

                                            2005022737

Indexing, Abstracting & Website/Internet Coverage

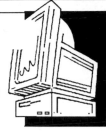

This section provides you with a list of major indexing & abstracting services and other tools for bibliographic access. That is to say, each service began covering this periodical during the year noted in the right column. Most Websites which are listed below have indicated that they will either post, disseminate, compile, archive, cite or alert their own Website users with research-based content from this work. (This list is as current as the copyright date of this publication.)

Abstracting, Website/Indexing Coverage . . . . Year When Coverage Began

- *Abstracts in Social Gerontology: Current Literature on Aging* **1993**

- *Alzheimer's Disease Education & Referral Center (ADEAR)* **1997**

- *Biosciences Information Service of Biological Abstracts (BIOSIS), a centralized source of life science information.* <http://www.biosis.org> **1982**

- *Brandon/Hill Selected List of Journals in Allied Health Sciences* <http://www.mssm.edu/library/brandon-hill/> **2000**

- *Business Source Corporate: coverage of nearly 3,350 quality magazines and journals; designed to meet the diverse information needs of corporations; EBSCO Publishing* <http://www.epnet.com/corporate/bsourcecorp.asp> **2003**

- *CINAHL (Cumulative Index to Nursing & Allied Health Literature), in print, EBSCO, and SilverPlatter, Data-Star, and PaperChase. (Support materials include Subject Heading List, Database Search Guide, and instructional video.)* <http://www.cinahl.com> **1980**

- *Developmental Medicine & Child Neurology* **1994**

- *EBSCOhost Electronic Journals Service (EJS)* <http://ejournals.ebsco.com> **2001**

(continued)

(continued)

* Exact start date to come.

Special Bibliographic Notes related to special journal issues (separates) and indexing/abstracting:

- indexing/abstracting services in this list will also cover material in any "separate" that is co-published simultaneously with Haworth's special thematic journal issue or DocuSerial. Indexing/abstracting usually covers material at the article/chapter level.
- monographic co-editions are intended for either non-subscribers or libraries which intend to purchase a second copy for their circulating collections.
- monographic co-editions are reported to all jobbers/wholesalers/approval plans. The source journal is listed as the "series" to assist the prevention of duplicate purchasing in the same manner utilized for books-in-series.
- to facilitate user/access services all indexing/abstracting services are encouraged to utilize the co-indexing entry note indicated at the bottom of the first page of each article/chapter/contribution.
- this is intended to assist a library user of any reference tool (whether print, electronic, online, or CD-ROM) to locate the monographic version if the library has purchased this version but not a subscription to the source journal.
- individual articles/chapters in any Haworth publication are also available through the Haworth Document Delivery Service (HDDS).

Healing 9/11:
Creative Programming
by Occupational Therapists

CONTENTS

ABOUT THE EDITOR

Pat Precin, MS, OTR/L, is currently the Managing Director of Pathways to Housing Inc., a housing-first, consumer-driven organization that provides scattered site apartments and assertive community treatment to chronically homeless individuals with mental illness and substance abuse. She has been the Director of the Brooklyn Bureau of Community Service's P.R.I.D.E. 2000 Program (Personal Roads to Individual Development and Employment), a performance-based Welfare-to-Work initiative that helps disabled public assistance recipients find and retain gainful employment. She has also directed the Occupational, Recreational and Creative Arts Therapy Programs at St. Luke's-Roosevelt Hospital in New York City. She is Adjunct Assistant Professor of Occupational Therapy at LaGuardia Community College and has directly supervised over 100 occupational therapy students in various clinical settings. Having eighteen years of clinical experience in the areas of psychosocial occupational therapy and substance abuse, she has authored three additional books: *Living Skills Recovery Workbook, Client-Centered Reasoning: Narratives of People with Mental Illness*, and *Surviving 9/11: Impact and Experiences of Occupational Therapy Practitioners*, and multiple journal articles and grants, as well as performed research studies in these fields. She serves on the Board of Directors for the following organizations: The Center for Community Integration, Inc., Housing First, Inc., The State University of New York Downstate Medical Center and LaGuardia Community College. She works actively with the Metropolitan New York State District Occupational Therapy Association (MNYD of NYSOTA) Mental Health Task Force. She has degrees in Biophysics, Psychology, Pre-medicine and Occupational Therapy and is a member of the following national honor fraternities: Tri Beta (Biology), Psy Chi (Psychology), and Mu Phi Epsilon (Music). Pat has been a long-term consultant for a consumer-run non-profit organization that guides mental health consumer entrepreneurs through their business ventures. She has spoken at international, national, and state conferences and at colleges and universities. She is also a published poet, musician, competitive athlete, photographer, and cave diver/explorer.

About the Contributors

Fran Babiss, PhD, OTR/L, is an occupational therapist who is the Program Director of an adult psychiatric partial hospital. On September 11, 2001, she was vacationing in Strasbourg, France. As a result, she made frequent trips to Ground Zero upon her return to New York, to validate that what seemed unbelievable had occurred. Photography and graphic arts are avocational pursuits, and her work has been published in books about French waterways as well as in this volume.

Donna Brennan is a freelance photojournalist for several New Jersey publications and newspapers and serves as a member of both the Fort Lee Film Commission and the Fort Lee Historic Committee. Donna's work on the film commission includes research and restoration of silent films made in Fort Lee during Fort Lee's days as the motion picture capital of the world. Donna also works with digital technology and production for public access programming, film festivals and retrospectives and the production of newsletters.

Joanne Cordero, OTR/L, is a staff occupational therapist in the Continuing Day Treatment Program at St. Vincent's Hospital in lower Manhattan. She is currently pursuing her Master's degree in Occupational Therapy at New York University.

Mary Beth Early has for 25 years taught in the occupational therapy assistant program at LaGuardia Community College, City University of New York. Her clinical experience has included inpatient psychiatry, community mental health, special education for children with emotional disorders, and long term care. She has practiced yoga regularly since 1976, is a long-time sustaining member of the Iyengar Yoga Institute of New York, and has studied Iyengar yoga with senior teachers in New York City, Berkeley California, and at the Ramamani Iyengar Memorial Yoga Institute in Pune, India. Her other interests include swimming, watercolor painting, and watching her son skateboard and play soccer.

Christina Forenz has an AS degree in Occupational Therapy from Rockland County Community College. She is currently a level II COTA on the SCI/TBI unit at Burke Rehabilitation Hospital.

Janine Gallo is a third year occupational therapy student at New York University working towards her master's degree. She is currently participating in her physical disabilities Level II fieldwork at Hackensack University Medical Center in Hackensack, New Jersey. Prior to attending New York University, Janine received her BA in psychology from Lehigh University in Bethlehem, Pennsylvania. Upon graduation from New York University, Janine will work for the New York City Board of Education in fulfillment of a loanship she was awarded by them. She plans to work in pediatrics and to possibly specialize in sensory integration therapy.

Corina Hall has a BS in Occupational Therapy from Utica College and is currently pursuing an advanced master's degree in Occupational Therapy at Bay Path College. She is an Occupational Therapy supervisor at the Burke Rehabilitation Hospital in White Plains, New York on the amputee, burn and orthopedic unit. She is also a frequent guest lecturer at Mercy College in New York.

Christina Hughes is the owner of a company called Transitions, which utilizes occupational therapy to assist people of all ages in finding their purpose in life through the venues of education and work. The goal of this business is to present individuals with practical tools so they are empowered to undergo often difficult, fearful transitions to achieve a higher quality of life. Christine is also a writer and is currently at work on her first novel.

Cheryl King began her career as a staff occupational therapist at St. Vincent's Hospital in New York City. For the past 24 years she has worked at St. Luke's/ Roosevelt Hospital Center (SLRHC) Department of Psychiatry, moving from clinician to supervisor to director of Occupational, Recreational and Creative Arts Therapy. For the past 6 years, Ms. King has served as the Clinical Systems Director, and Continuing Quality Improvement Director of the SLRHC Department of Psychiatry. Some of the many areas she has written and taught about during her career include: continuity of care for the chronically mentally ill, neurocognitive therapy in schizophrenia, occupational therapy treatment of borderline personality disorders, continuing quality improvement, and the use of humor in occupational therapy.

Jeanne E. Lewin is the author of Lewin, J. & Reed, C. (1998) *Creative Problem Solving in Occupational Therapy*, an interactive text. The publication is the first to introduce Creative Problem Solving, a thinking model that originated in the corporate environment, to health care. Jeanne presents Creative Problem Solving seminars and facilitates creative thinking to solve challenging problems in corporate environments. She is the founder and President of The Tramble Co. (www.tramble.com; Tramble@aol. com) (Frankfort, IL; founded in 1983) that provides learner-centered interactive workshops. Ms. Lewin also has an active clinical practice providing early intervention services to infants and their families. In 2001, she expanded her company to include multimedia production for creating web sites, web-based surveys, and video production services.

Dan Lynch has a BS/MS degree in Occupational Therapy from Dominican College. He currently is a level II staff therapist on the CVA unit at Burke Rehabilitation Hospital in White Plains, New York.

Chelle Marie, MSW, is Program Coordinator and Director of Job Development for the Brooklyn Bureau of Community Service's Community Response Center–9/11 Placement Program. She has developed, implemented, and directed numerous programs including an employment placement program for homeless families (Volunteers of America), an Assertive Community Treatment (ACT) program for individuals dually-diagnosed with psychiatric disorders and chemical dependency, a training program for mental health and substance abuse treatment professionals, a clinical research program (Department of Mental Health), and a continuing education program for licensed Social Workers (University of Georgia). She has conducted applied research in the areas of Welfare Reform, multi-modal treatment of psychiatric disorders, community integration of previously institutionalized, chronically homeless individuals, court-mandated parenting programs, barriers to employment among homeless single mothers, and she has assisted with research on Social Capital, Community Development, and Program Evaluation Guidelines for community service agencies while at Harvard University's John F. Kennedy School of Government. She has community development/famine relief experience working with war refugees in Swaziland, Africa.

Frank Pascarelli is a former firefighter, an Occupational Therapist with Children's Healthcare of Atlanta, and Advanced Rehab Services as well as a consultant on workplace and school violence prevention/intervention. He is also in the Air Force Reserves serving as a Biomedical Science Corps Officer with the 96th Surgical Operations Squadron at Eglin Air Force Base. He served during the Gulf War as part of a Combat Stress Control Team. Pascarelli was sent to New York to conduct a needs assessment and to provide crisis intervention in the post 9/11 period.

Mary Squillace BA, BS/MS, OTR/L, has been a practicing Occupational Therapist for seven years. Mary's teaching experiences include the creation and presentation of the seminar 'Reality 101' to graduating students, focusing on the transition from student life to practicing professionals; being an assistant professor at Long Island University for a practical anatomy lab; presenting and organizing seminars in Advanced Clinical Neurology for Touro College, the Manhattan Campus; teaching seminars in anatomy, kinesiology, physiology, emergency procedures, musculoskeletal injuries, and exercise programming for healthy people; and special populations seminars for the East Coast Instructor Training School associated with the World Fitness Alliance at various national sites. Clinically, Mary has worked at several medical centers located within the New York City and Long Island regions with a focus on traumatic brain injury, spinal cord injury and acute care. Mary is currently working within an outpatient care facility with a focus on hand therapy and home-based early intervention.

Joanne Torres is an Occupational Therapist who graduated from York College in 2002 and currently works as a Senior OT in Bellevue (with adults in a physical dysfunction setting). She lives on the Lower East Side of Manhattan and took a series of 9/11 pictures through her window that morning. Photography has always been her hobby and she particularly enjoys taking natural photographs.

Robert Young has a BS degree in Occupational Therapy from Worcester State College. He is currently a level II staff therapist on the SC/TBI unit at Burke Rehabilitation Hospital in White Plains, New York.

Christine Zimbelmann, MS, ADTR, CMA, is a registered Dance Movement Therapist and Certified Movement Analyst. She currently works in the continuing Day Treatment Program at St. Vincent's Hospital in lower Manhattan. She holds positions on the Boards of both the New York chapter of the American Dance Therapy Association as well as the New York Coalition of Creative Arts Therapists. In addition, she has a private practice in Dance Therapy and in clinical supervision.

Introduction
and Acknowledgments

Pat Precin, MS, OTR/L

Years after September 11, 2001, children nationwide experienced post-traumatic stress with symptoms of depression and anxiety as reported in *NYU Today*, 9/13/04 (pgs. 1, 4). Researchers concluded that watching the terrorist attacks on television or reading about them on the Internet or in the newspaper was sufficient enough to elicit these long-term symptoms. Children who had direct exposure to the event, in addition to the above, suffered also from separation anxiety and mistrust of others according to the report. Researchers recommended long-term interventions for the mental health reactions above and for substance abuse and aggression frequently noted in adults.

Healing 9/11: Creative Programming by Occupational Therapists is a follow-up to its predecessor, *Surviving 9/11: Impact and Experiences of Occupational Therapy Practitioners*, published by The Haworth Press, Inc. in 2003. Both books chronicle the experiences of OTs in their efforts to cope and heal in the aftermath of this disaster. *Surviving 9/11* focuses on the day of and shortly after the event, while *Healing 9/11* describes long-term interventions and programs established by OTs to aid children, firefighters, burn victims, psychiatric clients, students, displaced workers, and OTs themselves (Part I). It also describes the power of art and creativity in healing communities (Part II).

[Haworth co-indexing entry note]: "Introduction and Acknowledgments." Precin, Pat. Co-published simultaneously in *Occupational Therapy in Mental Health* (The Haworth Press, Inc.) Vol. 21, No. 3/4, 2006, pp. 1-2; and: *Healing 9/11: Creative Programming by Occupational Therapists* (ed: Pat Precin) The Haworth Press, Inc., 2006, pp. 1-2. Single or multiple copies of this article are available for a fee from The Haworth Document Delivery Service [1-800- HAWORTH, 9:00 a.m. - 5:00 p.m. (EST). E-mail address: docdelivery@haworthpress.com].

1

I would like to thank all the authors and photographers for their contributions to this book, Mary Donohue, PHD, OT, FAOTA and Marie-Louise Blount, AM, OT, FAOTA (Co-editors of *Occupational Therapy in Mental Health*), and The Haworth Press, Inc., all of which were integral in documenting OT interventions during 9/11. Additional thanks to Marilyn Maxwell and Peter LaBarbera.

FROM MY BEDROOM WINDOW: TIME-LAPSE PHOTOGRAPHY BY JOANNE TORRES

PHOTO 1.

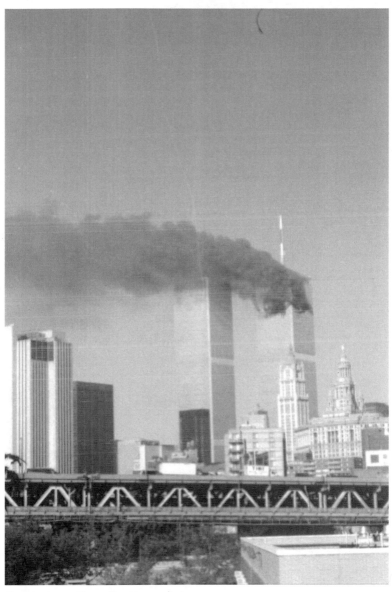

Photo by Joanne Torres. Used by permission.

PHOTO 2.

PHOTO 3.

PHOTO 4.

PHOTO 5.

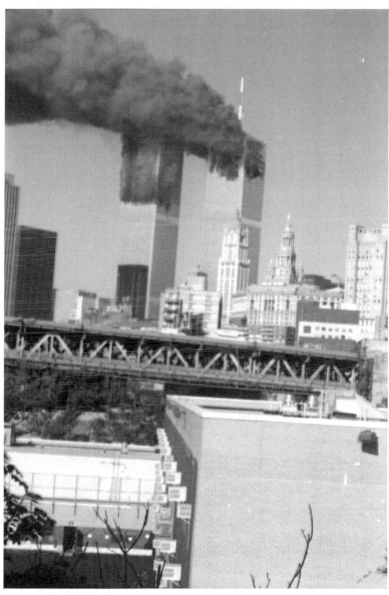

Photo by Joanne Torres. Used by permission.

PHOTO 6.

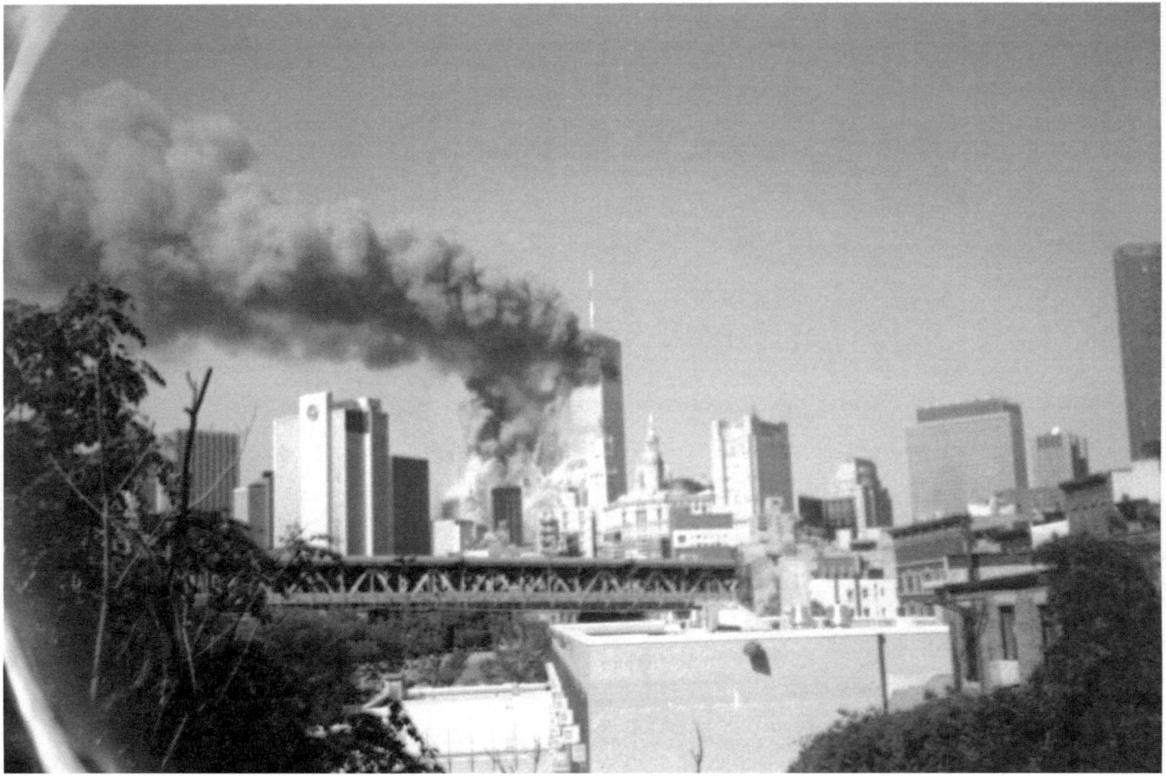

Photo by Joanne Torres. Used by permission.

PHOTO 7.

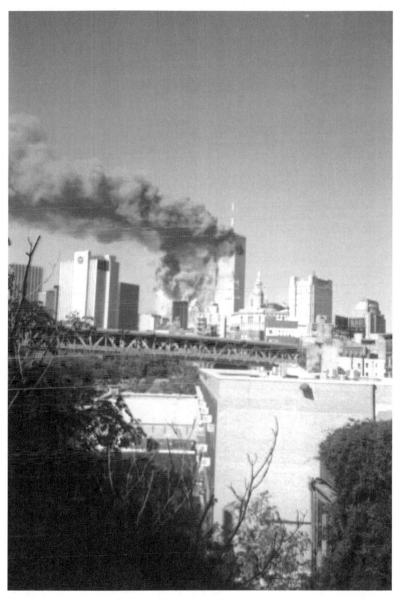

PHOTO 8.

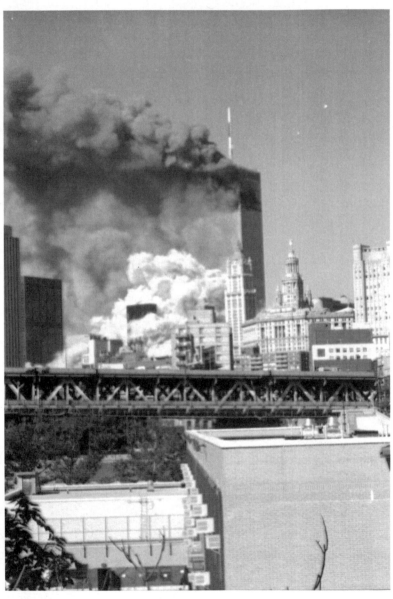

Photo by Joanne Torres. Used by permission.

PHOTO 9.

PHOTO 10.

PHOTO 11.

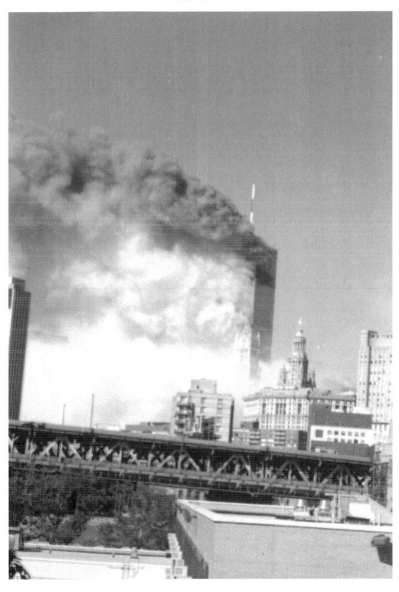

Photo by Joanne Torres. Used by permission.

PHOTO 12.

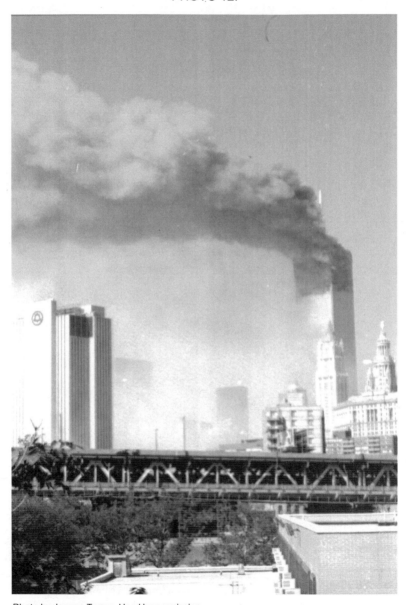

Photo by Joanne Torres. Used by permission.

PHOTO 13.

PHOTO 14.

PHOTO 15.

PHOTO 16.

PHOTO 17.

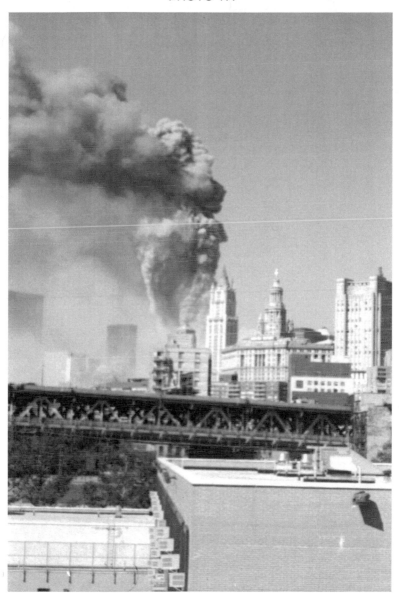

Photo by Joanne Torres. Used by permission.

PHOTO 18.

Photo by Joanne Torres. Used by permission.

PHOTO 19.

PHOTO 20.

PHOTO 21.

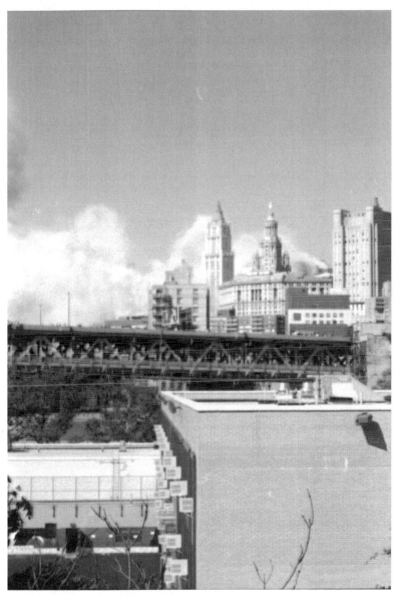

Photo by Joanne Torres. Used by permission.

PHOTO 22.

Firefighters.

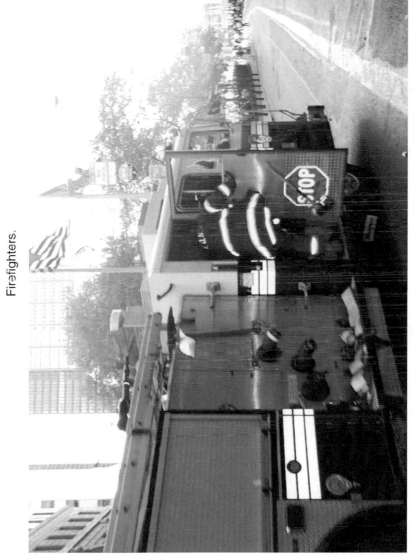

PART I:
PROGRAMS AND INTERVENTIONS

Counseling Firefighters Post 9/11:
An Occupational
and Dance Movement Therapists'
Interventions and Experiences

Joanne Cordero, OTR/L
Christine Zimbelmann, MS, ADTR, CMA

INTRODUCTION

In October of 2001, the Counseling Service Unit of the New York City Fire Department approached the administration of St. Vincent's Hospital, Manhattan, requesting help in providing outreach and counseling services to firefighters. At that time, the Counseling Service Unit or CSU had a staff of 11 full-time employees, consisting of psychiatric nurses, social workers, peer counselors, and firefighters who were retired or on light duty and reassigned to the CSU. With the events of 9/11 and the loss of 343 firefighters, the CSU was overwhelmed and inun-

[Haworth co-indexing entry note]: "Counseling Firefighters Post 9/11: An Occupational and Dance Movement Therapists' Interventions and Experiences." Cordero, Joanne, and Christine Zimbelmann. Co-published simultaneously in *Occupational Therapy in Mental Health* (The Haworth Press, Inc.) Vol. 21, No. 3/4, 2006, pp. 29-53; and: *Healing 9/11: Creative Programming by Occupational Therapists* (ed: Pat Precin) The Haworth Press, Inc., 2006, pp. 29-53. Single or multiple copies of this article are available for a fee from The Haworth Document Delivery Service [1-800- HAWORTH, 9:00 a.m. - 5:00 p.m. (EST). E-mail address: docdelivery@haworthpress.com].

Available online at http://www.haworthpress.com/web/OTMH
© 2006 by The Haworth Press, Inc. All rights reserved.
doi:10.1300/J004v21n03_02

dated by the needs of the members of the department and the family members of both the survivors and the deceased. Before September 11, the CSU handled about 50 new cases a month; by the middle of December 2001, it has opened more than 1,500 cases, and had visited and provided education to over 8,000 members of the Fire Department of New York (FDNY) workforce. They expect to see over 6,000 clients through private counseling, education, and group events by the end of 2002. Suddenly and without warning that 11-member team, which was more accustomed to handling isolated cases of alcoholism and grief was flooded with calls for its services. While the New York City Police Department held mandatory debriefing for all of its members, the FDNY adopted a slightly different approach. The FDNY implemented a more subtle method to address the complex needs of its members. This approach sought to both embrace and side step the insular, decidedly male culture in which firefighters tend to accept help only in the line of duty.

With regard to the department's approach to counseling and to mandatory debriefing, Dr. David J. Prezant, the Fire Department's Deputy Chief Medical Officer, stated in an interview for *The New York Times*, "If you go to people and say 'mandatory psychological counseling,' that hurts people . . . We're not going to do that. We're going to go to every firehouse and go time and time again. Whoever wants to talk to us, there's a counselor downstairs." In a "dominant male force with a lot of macho issues," he said, the challenge is getting across the simple message: "We are there for you" (Barry, 2001).

In terms of St. Vincent's collaboration with the CSU, seven staff members from the Department of Behavioral Health, which consisted of social workers, nurses, occupational therapists and a dance movement therapist, volunteered to participate in Project Liberty counseling services with the FDNY. Initially, teams of two St. Vincent staff were paired with one to two FDNY peer counselors with whom we visited various firehouses in the downtown area. Around the start of the year, a shift occurred and the St. Vincent's counselors "adopted" a house or two houses that they visited on a regular basis without the counselors from the CSU. Some of us from St. Vincent's worked individually and others in pairs.

GENERAL THEMES AND ISSUES

In counseling firefighters, some general themes and issues presented themselves. Some issues were present from the onset, some themes began to emerge over time, some have faded or resolved, and others have consistently reappeared session after session and continue to be present in the work. Some of the prominent themes and issues will be discussed in this section.

Treatment in the Workplace

Occupational therapists view treatment in the natural environment as enhancing the therapeutic process. It would seem a perfect fit that the therapists were accompanying the CSU peer counselors into the firehouses to provide treatment. However, as the first few sessions would demonstrate, this setup had its pros and cons, and at times it seemed the cons would outnumber the pros.

As each team of therapists would enter the firehouse, the procedure was basically the same. The person at the front desk, or house watch, would call the officer on duty. The officer, either a lieutenant or captain, would come to the front of the house to speak with the peer counselor. After a brief exchange explaining the purpose of the visit, if the men were available, an invitation to proceed to the kitchen would be given. (There was one instance when the session took place in the firefighters' quarters, or the room with beds where the men slept.) An announcement would come over the loudspeaker informing all the men to come to the kitchen. They would enter the kitchen and take their seats, either around the main table, or depending on the configuration of each kitchen, among the various seats available. In the ideal group setting, they would sit in a circle, where all members would be involved.

However, going into the firehouses, this ideal would not be the reality. Most houses had a large wooden table; in addition, many had additional tables and some had couches, chairs, or recliners, the type one would find in his/her living room. This would serve to be a problem as some would settle into these comfortable niches and engage in other activities such as reading the paper, resting with their eyes closed, or falling asleep. Other aspects of the physical environment not typically seen in a group session would be very much the normative in the firehouse. Attributes such as the physical space, the layout, the lighting, and the group room would vary but common things would be seen. For example, the lighting may not always be ideal. Some men would be hidden from view due to poor lighting.

This being their house, it would not be unusual for a visitor to arrive during sessions. These guests varied from some of the men who were stationed at the house but were passing through on their day off, were on leave and stopping by for a visit, or worked in that house previously but were now stationed elsewhere. This served to be a source of frustration as well as conflict. Could we be professional and ask the person to join in, or set a limit and ask the person to leave? Although we were there for a professional purpose, we were still guests as well, and often learned to work around these intrusions.

As the introductions and purpose of our visit was presented, some would be attentive and listen while others would continue to engage in their own activities, reading the paper, resting, or talking on the phone. This could be interpreted as a rejection of the visits, but another aspect to consider was that we were in their house and the activity did not stop just because we were there to provide group treatment. So the activity quieted down, the television would be turned off, people were attentive for the most part, but the phone would continue to ring, and the alarm, or the signal that they needed to respond, would continue to sound. This was perhaps the most frustrating and most analyzed aspect of this project. How could treatment be provided in this context? How could we ask these men to share their experiences, some very emotional experiences, as they would be expected to leave at the sound of the alarm to respond to a possible fire or other emergency? This is a definite disruption to any sense of a cohesive group process. However, there was no easy solution. There was no other way to reach these men other than to go into their place of employment. The likelihood of a firefighter coming into the counseling center was very slim. This was the only way to reach them and attempt to provide education, resources, and a forum to allow them to share their thoughts, feelings, and experiences.

Resistance

St. Vincent's was initially brought into the firehouses under the auspices of the CSU. The CSU of the FDNY has historically provided counseling services to men for personal, emotional, and mental health issues. When asked by the men, the CSU is commonly known for the treatment provided for persons with addiction issues, namely drugs or alcohol. As stated earlier, after 9/11, the CSU had to shift gears and respond immediately to the needs at hand. Individual treatment was made available. Numerous groups have been developed and offered to meet the various needs of the firefighters, their families and the loved ones of the deceased. There are currently groups for the grieving widows and families, the liaisons who worked with the families, and for survivors. However, the stigma that had been so closely associated with the CSU appears to have remained and may well be a factor in what is at times construed as resistance to the therapeutic process. As outsiders attempting to make our way in to this culture, we very much relied on and benefited from the education and insights of the CSU members when we worked together with them at the onset of this project. We might never have been accepted into the house without them. However, at the same time the stigma attached to the CSU may have contributed to the resistance. Many men have stated their distrust of the CSU. They feel fearful of their supervisors being informed of the fact that they have sought counseling and there is a fear that a change in duty status could possibly result.

During the early stages of being oriented to this project, we were told to anticipate the resistance of the men. As they say of those who help others, they are the ones who are most resistant to helping themselves. This is true of firefighters. During the initial sessions in the firehouses, we often asked the men, "How are you taking care of yourselves during this time?" Many of them would appear surprised by the question. Others would quickly answer, "I am not thinking of that right now"; "I do not know," or even "I am not " In the initial stages after 9/11, many of the men were in what they described as busy mode. They had experienced changes in their work schedules as they were asked to work 12-hour shifts. They were going down to Ground Zero to search for remains. They were attending funerals and memorials on their days off from work. Some attending even four to five memorials and funerals a day. Many houses were busy planning the traditionally elaborate funerals and memorials for their lost brothers. In addition, they were tending to the needs of the widow/families, not to mention their own families. Many men acknowledged that they had not been home, some for days at a time, and that they had little time for their spouses and children. Perhaps in order to maintain such an intense schedule and to keep up the pace they needed to defend against any painful emotions or acknowledgment of any weakness, vulnerability or suffering that they were feeling. We often asked ourselves, *"Are they resistant or are they sealing over for the time being in order to get through the day-to-day demands?"* Interestingly, many men made statements which indicated that they were concerned about or anticipated their own mental health being affected once all the frenzied activity died down, or "after the holidays," or "when there is no more digging at the site," or "after the last funeral/memorial." Perhaps, what we sometimes misconstrued as resistance was a necessary mechanism at the time.

As we continued to do this work even after the holidays, after the digging was complete, and the frenzied activity quieted a bit, we still encountered resistance to talking about certain feelings or experiences during some of the group sessions. This resistance was often on the heels of a warm polite welcome and the offer of a cup of coffee, and often some sort of baked item. We have spent a fair amount of time thinking about and discussing this among colleagues who are also doing this work. Resistance is common in therapy and most clinicians are familiar with it. We came to understand the resistance as a manifestation of strong cultural norms, long since established within the firehouse culture. The culture is primarily male dominated and many of its members struggled with the process of acknowledging a need or problem and subsequently accepting help. These men are in the business of rescuing others and are invested in maintaining a strong almost impenetrable exterior. As many of the men will tell you, the occurrences of the day within the firehouse along with any fires that may have been responded to, stay within the firehouse. Any discussion about firehouse activity is usually shared in the house as they sit around the kitchen table. We learned early on in this work that it is a common practice not to talk about the challenges or details of their work with loved ones. In fact, there is often a conscious attempt to conceal, guard and protect loved ones, even spouses, from the realities of the job. While this may serve an important purpose, it also perpetuates a dynamic in which there is an investment in not showing weakness, emotion or vulnerability, and in which open sharing and the receiving of support does not occur.

Is this resistance in the classic sense? One could argue that it is a necessary part of the job. With the occurrences of September 11 so widespread and the terror and destruction so readily seen in all forms of media, the spouses, significant others, family members and friends were now exposed to the events they had been protected and shielded from in the past. Naturally, they wanted to speak about what their loved one in the fire department experienced. Many of the men would say that they were not used to discussing details with those outside the job and this presented a conflict and put strain on relationships. The loved ones felt a natural curiosity. In addition they felt concern; and wanted to provide comfort and support. However, the details of what the firefighters had experienced were too gruesome and disturbing to share. So they tended not to talk about them; they shut down, pushed the experiences and memories aside, remained busy and strong, and denied their own vulnerability. As a result, many firefighters held these images and experiences inside.

Often this disinclination to speak about pain or suffering was apparent in our counseling sessions. Many were of the belief "Why talk about it; it does not change anything," or "Nothing we say can undo the situation or bring our brothers back." The idea that acknowledging feelings and giving voice to them may be valuable and help them to feel better was a new idea and was not altogether accepted. In some houses the men were able to talk about the fact that there was a stigma attached to anyone who sought out counseling. With regard to the need for but disinclination toward counseling services, one firefighter was quoted in the December 14, 2001 *New York Times* article, "Offering First Aid in a Firehouse Culture That Favors Toughness." He commented on what he observed to be "the quiet distress of some colleagues, the hollow look in their faces and stated, 'I don't think they have a clue. They're overwhelmed. And guys are going to tough it out. That's the attitude of firefighters.'"

Anger

Anger was one of the most prominent and palpable emotions displayed in many of the firehouses that we visited. Anger is a typical response to loss and is part of the grieving process. Many authors have suggested that the grieving process takes place in a series of stages. In most of the literature one of the early stages, after shock, denial, numbness or disbelief is anger. The bereaved can feel anger at the deceased for leaving them, at God for "taking" their loved one or allowing this to happen, or at the world in general for what often seems to be an inexplicable injustice. In the case of the World Trade Center attacks, many firefighters felt angry at being victimized, at the magnitude of the tragedy, at their own vulnerability and inability to prevent the loss of life or to rescue the victims, and at the mounting death toll of innocent people which included members of their immediate family, "brothers" from the job, friends, coworkers, mentors and leaders in the fire department.

Although these may have been the experiences and feelings the men were going through during this process, these were not the words they were speaking. The anger that was verbalized to us in the sessions was usually directed toward the FDNY administration, people on the outside, or even toward each other. There were some instances when we were informed that a particular house was experiencing increased fighting among its members.

Initially, this anger was often directed at Osama bin Laden, then at Fire Commissioner Thomas Von Essen and Mayor Rudolph W. Giuliani. The anger and rage was expressed during sessions at the firehouse, and at times became more public as in the case of a scuffle between a few members of the FDNY and a number of police officers that occurred at the disaster site after City Hall briefly reduced the number of fire-fighters assigned to recovering bodies at the scene. The fire department is a tradition-bound culture. A central idea and practice in their culture is that the job is not complete until everyone is saved or rescued and/or until all victims' bodies are recovered. The idea that someone from out-side the department, in this case the Giuliani administration, could dic-tate how and if the firefighters would be able to see this part of the job through to completion was the source of outrage among many of the men. I believe that in addition to inciting feelings of anger that the poli-tics involved compounded the existing feelings of helplessness, vulner-ability and guilt. Anger directed toward the job was prevalent as well. Many men described feeling more angry regarding long-standing prob-lems in the job such as low pay, working without a contract and use of inadequate or outdated equipment. In the aftermath of September 11, these issues became more inflammatory, yet few men, in my experi-ence, questioned whether or not to keep doing the job. They did, how-ever, at times question what to do with all their anger, especially considering that most of them felt that there was nothing they could do to bring about a change in its cause.

Loss of Control

The knowledge and skills a firefighter possesses that allow them to battle a blaze gives one a sense of control in the ability of man to tame the natural forces of fire. This sense of control has been shaken since 9/11. It was our sense that some of the issues that contributed to their an-ger stemmed from feelings of loss of control on multiple levels. There was a sense of vulnerability which all of America felt after the terrorist attacks. There was a sense of, *"How could this happen to us?"* due to the inability to foresee these attacks and the impending danger and anticipa-tion of another attack in the future. This feeling was intensified among the firefighters due to the magnitude of the impact on their brethren. One aspect they felt was in their control was to bring home their lost brothers. This was widely stated immediately after the attack. The FDNY would not rest until every lost brother was found and returned. This was the natural approach to take. Didn't they always bring home every man? However, due to the massive destruction, and interventions made by the administration this was not possible. The inability to bring home their lost brothers has added to the feeling of not being in control. As mentioned earlier, some of the limitations placed on the administration related to the number of men allowed to work at the site, the number of hours they could work, and a limitation on the time the site would be open for recovery to occur. These factors have severely impacted on their ability to bring home their 343 lost brothers and to give the families a sense of closure. This has not been an easy aspect for the men to accept and come to terms with.

Despite the widespread resistance, there were times during which the firefighters utilized our sessions as an opportunity to "debrief." They sometimes did this in the context of explaining something about the layout or engineering/design of the buildings, which would then lead to a discussion of what their own experiences had been like on that day. Numerous men commented on the fact that they had never seen such destruction or loss of human life, despite having been at hundreds of fire and accidents over the course of their careers with the department. Many firefighters stated that they had strong recollection of the smells and especially of the sounds that they heard on that day. It was often quite difficult to listen to the descriptions of these sights, smells and sounds. Several of the St. Vincent's staff doing this work experienced some degree of shared trauma as a result of hearing and absorbing these images from some of these rare sessions in which open and graphic sharing did in fact occur.

An important therapeutic message which was communicated from the beginning was that within the FDNY, no one was unaffected. For example, some men who were not at the World Trade Center that day spent weeks working on the recovery effort at Ground Zero. It was these men who often stated, "But I was not there that day," and tended to minimize the severity of their recovery tasks. However, these men were also traumatized as a result of their exposure during their efforts, and interventions were provided to legitimize their feelings. In the literature on PTSD, there is an assumption that the traumatic event occurred and is now in the past. The firefighters working at Ground Zero after 9/11 were exposed and re-exposed to traumatic events for weeks and months at a time. In light of this fact many of the treatment models designed for use with people suffering from PTSD were not relevant. The process of grieving, integration of experiences healing and moving forward was complicated by the nature of the event and by the nature of the recovery work done by our clients.

Substance Abuse

Another widespread issue that became evident in our counseling sessions was the increase in alcohol consumption. Often this topic was broached with the use of humor, and often during talk of how people were coping, handling the stress, and/or feeling good. While often masked by the use of humor, it was clear that for some firefighters this was a serious issue potentially leading to a serious problem. When we first started doing this work, men were still digging at the site 24 hours a day (Photos 1-2) and bodies were being recovered; remains were being identified on a daily basis. Many firefighters were attending funerals daily, and it was not uncommon to attend multiple funerals and/or memorial services in the same day. In many cultures, it is common to drink socially after a funeral or memorial service. It only follows that if firefighters were going to funerals daily for weeks at a time that there was the possibility of drinking daily whereas in the past alcohol consumption was far less frequent and less extensive. Firefighters will be the first to tell you that prior to 9/11 socializing in bars and winding down after a "tour" over a few beers was commonplace and part of their culture. Many firefighters stated that they were using alcohol to manage stress, help with sleep, bond with their brothers, feel good even temporarily and as a part of the ritual of burying and memorializing a fallen member of the department. Many men were not aware that alcohol is a depressant or that it actually interferes with sound sleep. Several firefighters mentioned the fact that their significant others had put pressure on them to decrease their consumption and others commented on the fact that the increase in alcohol consumption had contributed to weight gain, which was also a common phenomenon post 9/11.

Shift in Mindset, Belief System

An issue that has been discussed more recently centers on a questioning of the firefighters' core belief system. Traditionally there was an unwritten code of honor that each member would return from a fire alive because every brother looked out for all of the other brothers. But after 9/11 with the loss of 343 men, it was not possible to fulfill this aspect of the code of honor. Some have pondered and evaluated what their response might be should another catastrophe occur. Some have stated they would continue to serve in the line of their duty, whatever the outcome may be. Some have said that should another catastrophe occur, they would retreat immediately. Many have verbalized that they no longer feel fully confident in their skills and abilities as one man stated,

PHOTO 1. Men Digging in the Zone 24 Hours a Day.

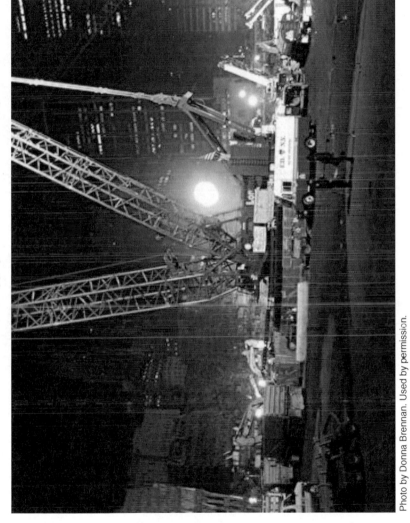

Photo by Donna Brennan. Used by permission.

PHOTO 2. Round the Clock Work in the Zone.

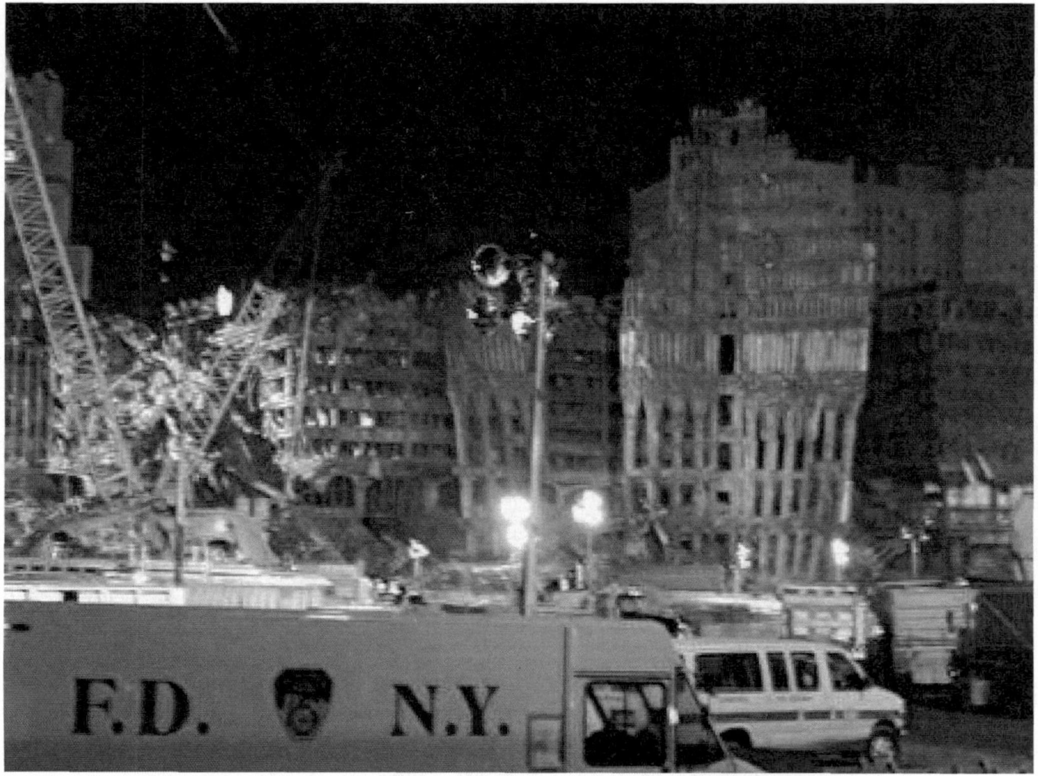

Photo by Donna Brennan. Used by permission.

"We do not just fight fires anymore." There have been discussions around a common feeling that their equipment is inadequate and antiquated. In addition, many feel that the administration has been lacking in their response to update policies and procedures, and to provide education and training which has not helped the problem. There has been some talk of a change in response for future catastrophes that the men would report to a neutral location and then be deployed from this location. There have been strong reactions to this. Many have felt that the administration intervening at this level would be ineffective. Some understand the thinking behind this as a means to control and monitor the number of men who respond. A factor which had been said to contribute to the enormous number of losses was the fact that many men who were not on duty responded to the World Trade Center and there was not an easy way to monitor or retrace the steps of many who were not working with their house that morning. But many feel this is in direct conflict with their natural calling. As one firefighter stated, "If that were your mother in that building, would you question if two extra men went in to rescue her?"

This shift has caused a rift in the camaraderie that was inherent and readily relied upon. A new mindset has emerged in that there is no guarantee that every man could be brought home. One firefighter made the analogy to the military as the next call may bring the unexpected and should that occur, the first few men to go down there would not be returning. This has been a disturbing thought for some. As they anticipate what the future holds, this has impacted on their fundamental beliefs. A firefighter who expressed a concern in the shifting mindset states, "I do not know what to expect during that call, if the man behind me really has my back, or will he retreat?"

An issue that seems to have recently emerged is the feelings that some of the firefighters have regarding their role in the public eye. This is both a complex and delicate issue and one, I believe, that it has been helpful to identify and explore during our sessions. Immediately following September 11, the firefighters were deemed heroes, and assumed a prominent role in the media and public eye. They became celebrities of a sort. Most of the men voice a deep appreciation for the outpourings of thanks and support, which they received from people all over the city, the country and the world. However, some expressed feelings of guilt regarding this "hero-worship." On more than one occasion I heard men make the analogy to the Veterans from Vietnam, saying, "Now those are heroes and what did they get when they returned home?" The war analogy came up frequently as men stated "we took this job to fight fires and rescue people, not to go to war." In the first months after 9/11, New Yorkers, Americans, and people from all over the world inundated the firehouses with food, cards, letters from people of all ages (Photo 3), artwork, memorabilia, tokens of love and support of all kinds as well as visits in person. While the intensity of all this has lessened with time, the visits continue. It seems as if the country needed to come to New York, down to Ground Zero and into a firehouse to hasten their own healing process. Often the visitors come to the house, at all times of day, often in groups, some bringing money they have raised from a local bake sale, plaques, T-shirts, and so forth. Perhaps doing so helps them feel like they have done something or repaid some debt. These actions do help people heal. However, the process of greeting the public day in and day out, answering questions and listen to people as they share their stories regarding September 11, often crying or breaking down themselves, has been incredibly trying and draining on the firefighters. It dawns on me that these men are doing counseling themselves for the general public. They welcome people into their house and listen patiently to their stories even in the midst of their own grief, their own struggle to resume some sense of normalcy and their own very busy workday. In our counseling sessions we have addressed the idea that anger and frustration at the general public is normal and have brainstormed techniques for dealing with this problem, as many of the men feel guilty for even voicing these feelings considering that most people who come to visit mean well.

Another newly-expanded role of the firefighters is that of family liaison. Historically when a firefighter is killed in the line of duty, the family of the lost firefighter is "taken care of." They are given financial support, emotional support and help with child rearing and projects around the house. Traditionally this assistance goes on forever. After 9/11, each house had several members who were designated as the family liaisons. These men have been overwhelmed by this new responsibility. Some have expressed uncertainty regarding what to say to the widows, how to talk to the families, having no formal grief counseling training. The other implication of this role is that the family liaisons often find it difficult to balance this responsibility with their own family responsibilities; often causing conflict within their own marriages, relationships and families.

CHALLENGES

Participating in this type of counseling proved and continues to prove to be quite challenging for the clinician. There are challenges on many

PHOTO 3. A Child's Wishes Two Weeks After 9/11/01.

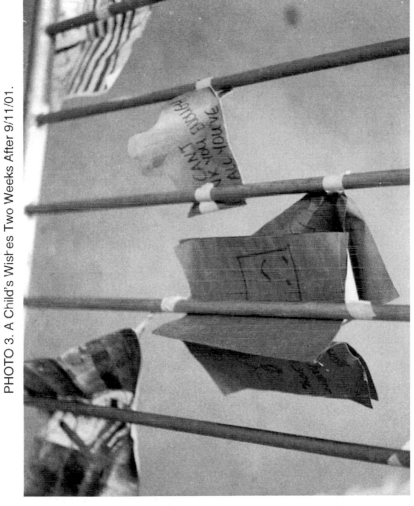

Photo by Barbara Ethan. Used by permission.

levels: personal, professional, logistical, and clinical. The following is a discussion of some of these challenges followed by a look at some of the treatment approaches and interventions utilized.

Disruptions to the Group Process

Inherent in the way our counseling sessions have been set up, there are both obstacles and benefits. The relatively simple task of arranging to go to the firehouse on a particular day and time has proven to be challenging, as it is impossible for anyone to predict what the workday might bring for a particular company. For example, the clinician might schedule a session for Tuesdays at 1:00 p.m. only to find that upon calling earlier in the day to confirm there is no one answering the phone or upon arriving at the firehouse that no one is at the house. It has not been uncommon for the clinician to make several phone calls before actually reaching a live voice and having to explain who we are and what we hope to do each time we want to schedule a session. It is also not unusual to be faced with the question of waiting until they return from a run, which can last anywhere from 15 minutes or several hours depending on the nature of the call. Assuming one gets in the door, the group counseling sessions occur in the kitchen of the firehouse. The clinician is in effect doing her work in the home of her client. Despite the fact that the purpose of the visit is to provide education and counseling, there is the element of being a guest and being treated as such, which cannot not be discounted or disrespected.

There have been times when the session is just underway or we have broached an important topic when the alarm sounds and the firefighters leap up and are on the rig and out the door. This also is not typical in traditional counseling situations. That having been said, there may be an adaptive function to some of the resistance to open sharing and expression of strong emotion and difficult subject matter. It has been a challenge to find the balance between trying to elicit expression and facilitate the debriefing process, while remaining cognizant of the need to function well in the event that they get called into the line of duty in the midst of the session. One of the initial challenges of this work has been establishing our role in the firehouse. As already mentioned, the fire department is a highly culture-bound organization. It is one in which its members take care of each other and is quite insular. As women, outsiders, and therapists, we did not have a natural niche in this culture, but had to work slowly and consistently over weeks and months to establish some sort of role in the firehouse. Several men have made reference to their discomfort speaking about their feelings or difficulties in front of a group, a group whom they know first hand has the potential to tease them mercilessly at any sign of weakness.

Unlike other treatment settings with varying client groups, the actual configuration of the firehouse group is different each time a session is held. Initially when we were doing this counseling with the peer counselors from the CSU, we might visit a different house each time we went out into the field. Over time as we revisited the houses, we started to get to know some of the men or at least see some familiar faces. As the work shifted and we were assigned a regular house or two, this became less of an issue. However the configuration of the group remains different on any given day, and this is not an element that one can predict or control. Thus the group dynamics are constantly in flux and it is difficult to follow up on an issue from one week to the next. Any continuity, trust or cohesion that may have been developed during a session does not progress and deepen in subsequent sessions. Thankfully and uniquely, the overall group cohesion, i.e., in the house itself, and the sense of trust and camaraderie between the members existed long before we ever walked in the door. This cohesion is an integral part of the workings of the house and of the firefighters' ability to function well and successfully do their jobs.

Establishing Role as Group Leader

Establishing our role as a group leader has been a challenge. In traditional group therapy, it is the group leader who establishes the group norms. However, when we were first oriented in preparation for this work, it was made perfectly clear to us that firefighters as a collective whole live and work as a group. They have clearly delineated and established group norms and group dynamics. Going into the firehouse, we had to be willing to veer from our typical way of working and not attempt to be the group leader, responsible for establishing the group norms. Instead, we had to be able to integrate ourselves into the pre-existing dynamics of the group. This is something that we had to learn over time during repeated visits.

Initially, it was necessary that the clinician play the role of guest and accept a cup of coffee, as it would be perceived an insult to refuse their offers of food and beverages. In keeping with this, it should be pointed out that as a group the firefighters are gracious hosts. Implicit in this setup is the notion that they are concerning themselves with the comfort and needs of the counselors before the attention and focus can be shifted onto their needs, feelings and experiences. As this was discussed earlier, they are comfortable in their role as helper.

Boundaries

As professionals working in a mental health setting, we are well aware of the need for boundaries due to the personal nature of the work we perform with our clients. The need to preserve our personal space, to protect our private lives and the importance of selective disclosure are aspects so inherent in our work. A shift has occurred for the clinician participating in this counseling work with the FDNY.

As mentioned earlier, entering into the house of these men one must play the role of a guest. In any traditional group setting, it is usually the group leader who gives to the group and the members who take from the group experience. There has been a necessary yet at times uncomfortable modification from the traditional boundaries that exist in any therapist client relationship.

In attempting to build rapport with these men, clinicians often find themselves being flexible with their boundaries in this setting. This often occurs in several ways. The therapist at times functions as a listening audience to some angry words, vulgar language, and some inappropriate humor at times. However, in order to be accepted where trust can develop, the clinician accepts the banter and attempts to subtly intervene or identify the real issue at hand. The clinician often has to ask a variety of questions of the firefighters, some personal (i.e., marital relations, eating, sleeping, and/or drinking patterns) and engage in personal discussions (i.e., travel commutes, the jokes about the administration and/or their nagging spouses) to participate in and stimulate discussion relating to how the men are coping, how the families are doing, and how they have been managing since 9/11. The clinician has had to wear different hats, some more uncomfortable than others. There have been times when they have engaged in heated discussions about the administration, or made negative comments about the CSU. Because we were brought into the houses through their administration and the CSU, it would not be appropriate to engage in these discussions, and yet setting a limit on these discussions would not be well received. However, they needed a forum to vent these frustrations. So, the therapist would allow them to express their feelings and attempt to address the underlying issues and ways to cope with their anger. Remaining neutral in response to some of the more public issues was difficult, often impossible, as we as citizens of New York and as Americans were responding to items in the news ourselves and as we began to feel connected to and protective of the firefighters ourselves. There have been a few instances when the tables have turned and the men have commented, "You have been asking us a lot of questions; how have you been coping?" In a traditional setting, a limit would be set as the focus is on the client and not on the therapist. However, this would not be the wisest intervention to make in the firehouse setting. We have often observed that if they are asking questions, then there is an interest or perhaps a personal concern about the issues being discussed. This was also an opportunity to provide a role model for positive coping techniques. So to facilitate further discussion, we have found ourselves talking about our own experiences, ways we have been coping, and sharing some personal information such as where we live and our marital status. This has felt awkward for us at times and was an issue, which each clinician has raised.

INTERVENTIONS AND APPROACHES TO TREATMENT

This was the first time we had ever done any counseling of this sort. There were no manuals or books written on how to do firehouse counseling in the wake of a devastating disaster of this magnitude. Often we did not know what to expect as we approached the session. In addition, all of us were dealing with our own personal losses, and reactions to 9/11. We did not approach this task with a unified, discrete treatment model or approach. Rather we utilized all of our clinical skills, intuition and experience working with trauma survivors and the bereaved. We tapped into our sense of humor and our deep desire to reach out and be of some help during a time when many New Yorkers and Americans were feeling helpless.

Flexibility is essential for participation in this project. As mentioned earlier, the challenges of going into their place of employment and attempting to provide group treatment is very different from conducting group treatment in the clinic setting from which we came. In the clinic, every group member comes voluntarily and is, generally speaking, there because they are willing to participate in the treatment process. It is a very different experience entering the firehouse. One has to be able to accept that the group formation and process is very different and will be different every time you walk in the door. The men in the group will be different and we have learned that with each grouping of men, the dynamics will be very different. There have been times when the clinician would enter the kitchen to find the men sitting around the table, and with minimal prompting, would participate willingly and share their stories, experiences, and frustrations.

Then there have been times when the clinician would sit at the table to find that despite the announcement coming over the loudspeaker, only one or two men would come into the kitchen, and preferred to engage in their own paperwork. The situations vary as often as the group configuration. Therefore, the clinician must be flexible and be ready to assess the group at the moment they come together and modify their approach accordingly. There may be times when the clinician will provide education, facts, and knowledge; other times the clinician will be a passive ear as the men share their experiences, vent their anger and frustrations, and hope to provide some interventions to address those issues. At still other times the clinician functions as "one of the guys," conversing with the group and engaging in jokes, bantering, and humor. The clinician needs to have a "bag full of tricks" for they never know what to expect. This need for flexibility and the ability to "go with the flow" without a set agenda parallels the process that occurs in a Dance Movement Therapy session. In that type, the therapist observes, meets the patients/clients where they are, and progresses from there toward the goals of the group. The idea of initially accepting and joining the client in whatever state they are in holds relevance to the firehouse work as well.

Realistic Expectations

With regard to expectations, the clinician who expects to conduct a group with every man sitting in the kitchen, ready, willing, and able to participate in a group discussion, is guaranteed to be disappointed and may easily construe this endeavor as unsuccessful. This is one aspect with which we were faced early on.

Every clinician has been faced with the various scenarios described previously, from the "perfect" group session to the sessions where the therapist felt as if he/she were "pulling teeth" and still not getting anywhere. As each group functioned differently and had varying needs, the clinician did not have a clear guideline for this type of work. As a result, initially, the clinicians struggled with the interventions they were making and questioned, *"Are we really helping these men?"* Each clinician adopted a different viewpoint. Some were discouraged and felt they were not being effective. Some were viewing this as a new endeavor and were open to whatever each experience brought. Early discussions with Frank Leto, administrative director of the CSU, brought some clarity. He stated, "Be small with your expectations." His viewpoint was that we were going in to provide whatever the men needed but there was no checklist for what they needed. So many of us reconfigured our agenda. A common format was that we would be going to the houses on a regular basis to provide consistency, a forum for the men to share their experiences, education to clarify and normalize their experiences, and information about additional resources at St. Vincent's for those who felt the need to reach out. The factor that we all had to keep in mind was that for many of these men, talking and accepting help would not be easy. Hence, for some, myself included, at times my expectations were as small as "Hey, they let us into the kitchen."

Education/Acceptance

One of the main goals in this work is to provide education regarding common reactions to a traumatic event or loss. We often focused on providing psychoeducation and reassuring the firefighters that what they are feeling and experiencing are "normal" and that they were not "crazy." We found that this was most effectively accomplished when we used non-clinical terms and tried to help the firefighters to accept that they were in most cases having strong but very normal, typical reactions to a traumatic event. Some of the main reactions that we consistently alerted the firefighters to be on the lookout for were the following: feelings of intense loss, grief, anger and rage, fear, hopelessness, irritability, numbness, having outbursts of anger, anxiety, having recurring dreams, distressing dreams or memories, having flashbacks, being more forgetful, having difficulty concentrating, and physical reactions (rapid heart rate, rapid breathing, difficulty sleeping, startling easily, hyper-vigilance, jumpy, and nervous). We also have been encouraging anyone who has been having prolonged acute stress reactions, still is not feeling any better, is having marital difficulties, substance abuse, and/or ongoing sleep interruptions to seek individual treatment and in some cases a psychiatric evaluation. One of the most critical approaches or interventions that we made has been to provide acceptance, to avoid pathologizing the behaviors and to provide support and reassurance. In the majority of cases simply being aware of the expected responses, being reassured that they will most likely begin to feel better over time, or having a few individual counseling sessions has helped tremendously. During sessions, we often speak about ways to cope with the reactions, emotions and stress that are occurring.

In one session, the main focus was on what would prompt one to reach out for help, what would allow a man who needed it, to pick up the phone or to go for help. No one could easily answer that question, but they were able to identify some of the barriers to reaching out for help. Inherent in this male dominated culture was the idea that men are strong; they cannot display any weakness. But in addition to this, there was the fear of their superiors finding out or of a change in their duty status occurring if they sought out help. The therapists focused on the available resources outside of the CSU, of the availability of staff at St. Vincent's where anonymity would be preserved. The emphasis was not on seeking counseling, but rather clinicians were available if anyone had any questions, just wanted to meet with someone to talk to, to ask questions, or for support. There was a strong emphasis on the fact that if they decided to speak with staff, their visit would remain anonymous, the CSU would not have to know about it, and their duty status would not be affected. A seemingly simple statement was made about the anonymity of our voice mail system, that if a message was left for a particular therapist, only that therapist and only that therapist would have access to that message. The response was interesting because in our jobs, we are mostly in group sessions, at meetings, or completing chart work; rarely are we at our desks. It is also rare that someone would catch a therapist "live" on the phone. So to state the obvious was an effective intervention. Some of the men seemed comforted by the fact that even if they did not get the person live on the phone, it was okay to leave a message because it would only be retrieved by that therapist. At the end of the session, there was one man who stated, "Oh, you will be getting a phone call from me."

Occupational Therapy Interventions

If asked about the occupational therapy interventions, one cannot clearly articulate what specific interventions or treatment approaches are used. Upon further discussion and evaluation of our work with the FDNY, some of the interventions can be identified but their implementation has occurred on a smaller, subtler scale. It seems as though the specific skills that are inherent in the therapist are conveyed on a subconscious and subtle level. For example, in the early part of our work, many of the men would describe the changes in their schedule due to the long hours they were working, attending numerous funerals and memorials, addressing the needs of the widows and families, and the effects on their families. For Joanne, the occupational therapist, the issue of time management was identified. However, in providing an intervention, one could not say, "*It looks like you have an issue with time man-*

agement." Many of the men simply accepted this as their responsibility and proceeded with these tasks as being necessary during this time. Many recognized that their wives and families were getting the short end of the stick. Some had the attitude that "They are just going to have to deal with it." There were very different responses and attitudes in this aspect. Attending the funerals and memorials seemed to be a common source of stress and conflict. Generally, when a firefighter had fallen in the line of duty, the funeral would be attended by all of his brothers with all the traditional finishes of a firefighter's funeral. Prior to 9/11, the FDNY would average one to two funerals a year. With the magnitude of losses among the FDNY, this average had increased 300 fold. Funerals being very emotional events, it goes without saying that attending three, four, or even five in one day would be overwhelming for anyone. Some of the men were able to verbalize feeling burned out from the multiple and seemingly never ending funerals, memorials, and subsequent funerals after a memorialized brother was found. Many people felt conflicted; they were emotionally exhausted from these events, but yet felt compelled to attend because that was the tradition. So to simply chalk it up to a time management issue was not the only aspect of this complex issue. An approach that was taken was to acknowledge that this was their tradition; however, with the sheer magnitude of this catastrophe and the numerous funerals and memorials, the men were asked to consider taking care of themselves and to set some limits if they felt overwhelmed. But in saying this, we did not know if that would be acceptable; that was another issue. It seemed that in some houses, some of the men were given flack if they had not attended their fair share of funerals. But what was considered a fair share? There was no easy way to address this issue or to intervene in any organized approach utilizing a particular frame of reference or theory. It was important to encourage them to give themselves and each other "permission" not to attend every funeral and memorial service.

In discussing this project, Christine also recognized that her skills as a Dance Movement Therapist were applicable here as well. Upon reflection of our work, she recognized that she was attentive to their level of physical activity and almost always emphasized the importance of physical activity and exercise in relation to stress management, anger management, when the opportunity presented itself. Many men reported that generally they do exercise regularly but that since 9/11, they have been unable to maintain this important part of their self-care routine. We encouraged them to resume some sort of regular exercise or physical activity even in the midst of all their other responsibilities.

Consistency

At this stage in our work, each therapist or team of therapists has now been assigned to one or two houses to which they visit on a regular basis. It is the hope that with consistent, regular visits, the men will begin to recognize the therapists, become familiar with them, and should the need arise, feel comfortable enough to approach them and seek help if needed. In the early stages of our work, several men in a variety of houses commented on the number of "good Samaritan" therapists, counselors, and outreach workers, who visited the houses to provide counsel and support. Some found them helpful only to realize that they were only in New York on a temporary basis and soon left to return to their home base. One man commented, "There was this one therapist who said she would return. She only came once and never came back." These experiences have been a source of disappointment, frustration, and anger. Some expressed anger at feeling like "targets," feeling overwhelmed by the number of "do-gooders" but none that seemed invested for the long haul. There was frustration at the numerous professionals who were all coming in to help. So, what makes us any different? At first, we were not sure. However, at this stage, we have been able to recognize the frustration of the men with these visits, but have emphasized that we are assigned to the house for a particular day and time and will continue to show up as long as they let us in the door. For most of us, we are still in the early stages of developing a bond with our "adopted" firehouses, but we are slowly starting to see some of the same faces, and those men are starting to see our faces. We are receiving some more receptive hellos, and some men who have stayed silent in the past are slowly starting to comment and participate. There was one who said, "All right, you have gotten me to talk." So for now as we work with our adopted house, it appears that providing consistency and regularity has been effective. It is our hope that should a need arise in the future, or should another event occur, a resource will be in place, a readily accessible and trusted resource.

This work remains unpredictable and changeable. As the anniversary of September 11 approaches, we notice a range of reactions. Some men have articulated feeling tense anticipating that day; not knowing what to expect or how they will feel. Some question, "Shouldn't I be 'over this' by now; it's been a whole year?" Others who may not have been stable are clearly feeling worse as the anniversary approaches and the reality of the event and the losses sink in. We continue to stress that each person's process is unique and to provide ongoing guidance and support.

As the clinicians, we forever question and evaluate our effectiveness in this project. We struggle with our own resistance at times and recognize that perhaps we have made a dent in the stigma regarding what it means for the firefighters to engage in the counseling process, however loosely we have defined that process. It has been the most challenging, yet uniquely rewarding work of our careers.

REFERENCE

Barry, D. (2001, December 14). Emotional first aid in a firehouse culture. *New York Times.*

Overcoming All Odds

Corina Hall, BS, OTR
Christina Forenz, AS, COTA
Dan Lynch, MS, OTR
Robert Young, BS, OTR

CHRISTINA FORENZ

For myself, the morning of September 11 began as usual. I was first informed about the World Trade Center attacks at 9:30 AM as I entered a room that was filling with patients for a group. All at once, every person began telling me about what had been happening for the last 45 minutes. Most of the patients had been getting ready for program or eating breakfast as every station on television suddenly interrupted their scheduled programs to broadcast the horror unfolding. Many witnessed the second tower being struck while they watched news reports on the first plane crash. It was difficult to continue with the group, as I also wanted to watch the news. For hours, the only information I received was via patient and staff report. I remember many staff members trying to locate family and friends in hope of good news and their safety.

My initial response was disbelief and hope that no one I knew would be involved. Around lunchtime, I was finally able to access a television to watch some of the coverage. The scene and the chaos going on, not only at the World Trade Center, but also within the entire city, as well as

[Haworth co-indexing entry note]: "Overcoming All Odds." Hall, Corina et al. Co-published simultaneously in *Occupational Therapy in Mental Health* (The Haworth Press, Inc.) Vol. 21, No. 3/4, 2006, pp. 55-64; and: *Healing 9/11: Creative Programming by Occupational Therapists* (ed: Pat Precin) The Haworth Press, Inc., 2006, pp. 55-64. Single or multiple copies of this article are available for a fee from The Haworth Document Delivery Service [1-800- HAWORTH, 9:00 a.m. - 5:00 p.m. (EST). E-mail address: docdelivery@haworthpress.com].

doi:10.1300/J004v21n03_03

across the United States, was almost unbelievable. As these images were shown over and over again, it was difficult to return to work. Though many people perished in the attacks, I knew there would be those who sustained injuries and I wondered if anybody would be admitted to Burke for rehabilitative needs and if so what would their injuries be. In November, the hospital admitted its first Word Trade Center survivor followed in the upcoming weeks by three more patients, all with extensive burn and pulmonary injuries.

There were many Occupational Therapy and personal challenges I had to face with these patients arriving at Burke. Gaining the patient's trust was a challenge although it seemed to have been obtained quickly. Burke, never having been known exclusively for treatment of burns to such a degree, required therapists on the unit to stand up to the test and show what we were capable of. Prior to treating these patients, I had little Occupational Therapy experience with such extensive injuries from burns. When we learned that we were receiving these clients from Cornell, therapists from Burke were sent to Cornell to observe the clients' current treatment of the massive hand and upper extremity injuries that the clients had incurred. I was informed that I would be assigned to one such patient, Lauren, along with a registered Occupational Therapist, as primary therapist. I began reading materials sent from the head therapists at the Cornell Burn Center along with textbooks containing information regarding burns, and appropriate treatment. Forced to learn quickly made treatment challenging, however, well worth the effort. Through our willingness to learn, we would gain the trust of Lauren to provide all the care needed for her recovery process. Many of the staff at Burke spent extra hours to learn treatment techniques with manual therapy, wound care and scar management from the therapists at the Cornell Burn Center. Communication between the therapists at the two centers was ongoing and of great assistance to all involved.

The World Trade Center victims challenged us emotionally during their entire stay at Burke. This was evident during every treatment session, proof that Occupational Therapists were not only capable of treating the physical/functional aspects of a patient's recovery but also addressing the psychosocial/mental needs. Lauren made me cry, made me laugh, and showed me that I could still have great fun even during the lowest and worst moments of life. Fluctuating moods from Lauren, ranging from happy to sad, and everywhere in between also presented a challenge and sometimes we saw a range of emotions within a treatment session. The personalities of each of the survivors being treated were unique. I have mentioned to Corina, our supervisor, that she could not have managed to pair therapists with patients any better. Though many Occupational Therapists treated these special patients throughout their stay, the primary therapists assigned were a perfect match.

Time became a factor when treating the Word Trade Center victims. They received Occupational Therapy for three-plus hours a day. With so much to work on, eight hours a day would not have been enough; thus two therapists were assigned to each burn patient. The staff put in many extra hours during the rehabilitation of these patients. Treatment for each patient consisted of manual therapy, range of motion, wound care, splinting, strengthening and activity of daily living retraining. My vision of Lauren when I first met her would be a woman who was very weak, de-conditioned, slow moving and passive. My vision was wrong! Lauren was a strong, vital woman, determined, humorous with a take-charge attitude, and yet still vulnerable to her injuries and emotional state. One of my most memorable treatment sessions with Lauren was when she wanted to work on applying makeup; she was determined to do so independently. My supervisor suggested I take Lauren to Bloomingdale's for her first community skills outing to work on this goal. Lauren would practice everyday skills of coordination while beginning her re-integration into society after being in the hospital for four months. Lauren was ecstatic and stated how normal it felt to be out in public. She never thought her disfigured appearance from the burns was abnormal, a true sign of her determination. Lauren applied her makeup diligently with much difficulty and compensation, however she had done most of it on her own. Her independence was a symbol of positive things to come. She was so happy to look and feel more like the beautiful woman she was before the injuries.

Therapists were challenged to balance their relationships with clients between therapist and friend. We all became close to our clients but were able to maintain the control needed to provide therapeutic interventions. The friendship part of the relationship came after the therapy. Lauren invited Corina and me to accompany her to an awards dinner in which she was being honored for her bravery and determination. We decided it would be appropriate for us to join her for this event. This would be the first time Lauren had been downtown since the collapse of the towers and she seemed to maintain a sense of calmness during the drive down, although it shocked her as to why so many of the streets were still shut down in lower Manhattan. She had been working on her therapy so intensely that she had not envisioned the massive destruction of property that was still being cleared away and sifted through. At the awards dinner that night, Lauren, ever so gracious, received the loudest and longest applause of all those being honored that night. She was truly a hero and a symbol that we are all survivors, no matter what the circumstance.

There were many rewards personally and professionally for me during and after treating Lauren at Burke. The primary surgeons and doctors from the burn center had commended us for the care and treatment given to Lauren during her rehabilitative stay. Her primary doctor here at Burke was commenting continually on the hard work and dedication we brought to the treatment. Lauren always told us we were rebuilding her body and would give us credit for her progress and all we had done for her. Besides the recognition from clients' families and colleagues, I feel the best recognition came from knowing how these individuals arrived at Burke and how they left. They were able to return to many of the roles they had assumed prior to 9/11, and I knew that I had made a difference to their functioning. Lauren and I have maintained communication since her discharge from Burke. We have developed a bond that will never be broken.

DAN LYNCH

It becomes a challenge in everyday practice to demonstrate empathy without sympathy for the consumers of your services. This professional behavior allows the practitioner to maintain his/her objectivity and provide treatments that are necessary. For example, the survivor of a stroke has suffered the loss of significant function and the etiology of this loss is well known. While the Occupational Therapist can provide support and compassion for the individual with full knowledge of the precipitating factors, which has brought this individual to professional services, the rapport between the therapist and the patient is based upon current interactions and is not clouded by a personal history. Difficulties arise when the practitioner has a shared history with the patient, especially one with the degree of emotions connected to the events of 9/11.

The 9/11 events have impacted all Americans in one way or another, whether it be the wife who lost her husband on that day, the child whose father was injured, or the mother who now fears for her child's future. Regardless, these events created a national sense of family and personal history. With this in mind, the therapist who works with a survivor of these events is put in a somewhat difficult situation in that the precipitating factors which brought this individual to professional services has also impacted the practitioner. The professional distance, which allows therapists to maintain their objectivity, has been decreased.

A client/therapist relationship lacking professional distance can affect the type of interactions and interventions given to the clients. Examples from the in-patient rehabilitation unit at our facility include frequency of treatment and the type of encouragement provided to these clients. At any given point in the day, many clinicians would offer additional treatment time and opportunities to victims of 9/11. In addition, many of the therapists were known to stay at work for up to two hours longer than their normal day in order to provide additional treatment and family education, and to fabricate/modify splints and other therapeutic media. This in no way infers that these individuals should not have been provided with such opportunities, however the motivation for these actions may have been influenced by a decrease in professional distance inherent in the relationship. This type of relationship additionally influenced the manner by which many therapists interacted with these World Trade Center patients. Clients' occasional lack of motivation and noncompliance with their exercise programs and activities provided on the unit were not addressed the same way for 9/11 victims as they were for the other patients. Encouragement was provided with caution as opposed to enthusiasm in an effort to protect or cause no further emotional harm to the victims of 9/11 who had already suffered so extensively. Albeit in hindsight, the fact that these patients were able to cope with what they had endured should have cued us as clinicians to their resilience as opposed to frailty.

In addition to the internal struggle of balancing professional responsibility and personal feelings are the expectations for recovery, which inevitably ensue from external sources. The events of 9/11 were covered extensively by the media, and in turn, the rehabilitation of these individuals at our facility was a matter for public consumption. On any given day, media outlets from newspapers to television magazine programs would be present to witness treatment and conduct interviews. There seems to be a pervading sense in our culture that all things connected to these tragic events belong to the masses, including the rehabilitation of these survivors. It was not long before strangers on the street would stop and ask for updates on patient progress, based on some information gathered from newspaper articles. This raised an interesting ethical issue for Occupational Therapists. Because confidentiality is always a concern, the clinician acknowledged the support generated by the public without disclosing personal information about any one client.

In the context of abundant and continued media coverage and the pervasive nature of the events of 9/11 in daily life, facilitating the ability of the survivors to develop health and appropriate coping responses provided a significant challenge. Occupational Therapists have a unique opportunity within the medical model to assist survivors of traumatic events towards developing healthy strategies and responses to stressful circumstances. The development of these strategies ultimately allows the survivor to obtain closure of the event and optimism toward the future. The process of obtaining this closure is significantly hindered by constant reminders and attention given to an event that the survivors required some degree of distance from. Fostering interests, engaging the other facets of the individual's life, and promoting independence in activities of daily living, met this challenge. The process of engaging the survivors of 9/11 in normal life proved to be the most effective strategy in that the rest of the world seemed quite occupied with how they were dealing with the event when in essence, they needed to deal with the aftermath of normal life. Above and beyond all physical agent modalities and advanced manual therapy techniques, the most useful therapeutic medium was the basic underlying tenet of occupational therapy practice itself, engaging in normal life.

ROBERT YOUNG

On 9/11 I was upset after hearing about the towers, but was devastated from watching the news that day and evening. It truly felt like I was watching a movie and that all the death and destruction was not a reality. I wondered how I could help these people, and I wondered if any of the injured would be admitted to Burke for rehabilitation. In November, the first of four burn patients arrived at Burke. My supervisor, Corina, was the victim's primary therapist and had asked me to assist with his range of motion. I was very gentle and careful, using great caution to not injure him. Corina said it is all right to be more aggressive but with the patient in pain during this stretching process, I felt bad for inflicting more pain, even if it was for his own good and recovery. I asked Corina if I could be the primary therapist for the next burn patient arriving at Burke, and she said that I would be assigned to Lauren. We were fortunate to have the opportunity to go down to the Cornell Burn Center together prior to Lauren's arrival at Burke and interact with her and her Occupational Therapist as well as observe critical treatments she was receiving on her hands. We arrived at the Burn Unit and were given an update on Lauren's status, with her Occupational Therapist stating that she was burned over 80 percent of her body and had extensive skin grafting. I started to feel some anxiety inside, asking myself the question, *"Will I be able to fill the role needed to care for a patient with such extensive burns?"* Prior to entering Lauren's room, I pictured a bed with a quiet, introverted patient who would take the role of the sick patient with control given to all medical personnel. Lauren certainly did not fit that role. She was very extroverted, independent with stating her needs to all disciplines, and was in complete control. Lauren was very talkative and was getting ready for a film crew to take footage for the "Oprah Show." My anxiety increased when Lauren told her Burn Center Occupational Therapist that she had nothing against us at Burke, but she had some reservations against going to a hospital that is not known for its burn care. We reassured her that most of her treatment was all in the realm of what we do with any other patient, with a few extra components. It was hard for me personally to reassure her as to my skills because my experience was limited to time as a student. I was surprised to see Lauren walk a long distance to the elevator and to the Occupational Therapy clinic. She sat down, put her hands on the table, and was ready to begin. I was surprised at how aggressive the stretching and manual therapy was to her hands and was told that it was necessary. My pen could not write quick enough to keep up with all the instructions that I was receiving regarding Lauren's treatment plan.

From the minute Lauren arrived at Burke, I felt it was important to educate staff on what I had learned at the Cornell Burn Center, and from my past experience and research. I had the opportunity to train nursing staff working with Lauren as well as my colleagues in the Occupational Therapy Department. Burke also accommodated us by bringing in experienced burn therapists to lecture and give hands-on training to those working with Lauren. From these lectures I learned that many standard Occupational Therapy treatments used on orthopedic and neurological patients could be applied to and were acceptable treatment for burn patients. For example, prior to these lectures, I would never have expected that a thermal modality, such as paraffin, could be used on a burn patient.

Early in Lauren's treatment, she would be shuddering from the pain that was involved with her aggressive manual therapy. As a therapist, I had trouble putting a patient through such pain at first and made sure she received pain medication prior to our treatment sessions. The medication helped, along with Lauren practicing meditation, counting and breathing techniques. After a couple of weeks, her routine became more tolerable for both of us. Treatment did not always have pain associated with it. It was beneficial for Lauren to be distracted with conversation and laughter. On the weekend after completing range of motion on her hands, I would pretend her joints were like a creaky door at a haunted house. We could not stop laughing. The weekends were a time to focus her treatment on interacting with her 14-month-old son because he was only allowed to visit on the weekends. This involved holding and playing with him. Family education was also an important component, and again the weekends lent themselves to this type of training. Lauren and I would also have fun dancing in her Occupational Therapy exercise group with a focus on range of motion and stretching. I had very high standards for Lauren. It was a challenge for her to wear splints every moment that she was not actively using her hands. I know Lauren was capable of being pushed hard and she would always give her all with managing her splint schedule. Lauren gave nothing less than 110 percent throughout her treatment. At times we would disagree and argue, but after discussion, we usually reached a mutual agreement about her care. I have to admit I was not quite used to someone who wanted such control of her own medical treatment. The majority of patients say, "Tell me what to do next" or "I do not know, you are the expert," when trying to form goals. It was a new experience to have a patient say, "I will do this."

Ultimately the time came for Lauren to be discharged home. Her leaving was difficult. We had spent over three months together as therapist/patient as well as friends. I had developed a relationship not only with Lauren, but her husband and son as well, and I would miss them all. I was lucky in that I knew she would be back to visit and we would get together on a regular basis to catch up on her progress and her life back in her home environment. I will never forget the impact Lauren had on me as an Occupational Therapist and as an American. Lauren had a spirit about her that will stay with me throughout my professional career and that I will always cherish.

CORINA HALL

My first thought about 9/11 today and on the actual day is what a beautiful day it was, a cloudless blue sky and bright sun, the total opposite of ominous events to come. I perceived the events of September 11 as unrealistic or something that only happens in other countries, certainly not ten miles away from my backyard. But there we were, faced with devastation and death that we as Americans are not accustomed to. The chaos in Manhattan that day was incomprehensible. Imagine, New York City, shut down, with everyone trapped. Colleagues were in a constant state of uncertainty, as calls could not be made to loved ones to find out if everyone was all right. As an American, I felt violated as we were robbed of two structures that represented our country almost as significantly as the Statue of Liberty.

As days went on, I was desperate to lend assistance. My only hope was that victims would come to Burke and I could meet their rehabilitative needs. I first heard of burn patients being admitted to Burke in November. Being the supervisor, I was asked by admitting doctors here if we were equipped to meet the needs of these severely involved victims. As is my usual style, I said "absolutely" before considering all the factors involved in burn rehabilitation, but I also knew this was not an opportunity to be passed up. Many of my colleagues were feeling as helpless as I and this was a chance to redeem our spirits and hopes, and show our true colors as therapists and rebuilding function into the lives of these chance survivors.

I became the primary therapist for Harry, a quiet, intelligent man who was burned on approximately 40 percent of his body, with the most extensive damage to his face and upper extremities. I was prepared for completing his physical care and treatments, but was not prepared for the emotional component I would feel whenever working with him. It is very challenging to separate emotions from professional behavior because as a therapist you needed that component of compassion to assist the patient in overcoming simple daily obstacles. I kept thinking, *"This was a man who was a respected professional, wonderful husband and father, and now at times lay helpless and in so much intense pain that I felt inadequate."*

In addition to my own internal struggle, we were receiving more burn patients and I had to rally my colleagues to put forth a confident and assertive appearance. I pulled myself together and began educating my staff in manual therapy techniques, adaptive devices and splinting needs that would need to be met for each patient. There were also the never-ending tasks of keeping wound care supplies, treatment modalities, and references at everyone's fingertips. And where would we all find the time needed to complete all treatment, educate staff and family and maintain the high level of care we offer to all patients that come through our doors here at Burke? The balancing act for me was the biggest challenge because we all wanted to spend our free time helping 9/11 survivors. We sought solace in each other as therapists to relieve ourselves of frustration and to problem solve as a team on treatment plans and strategies. As a supervisor, I noticed that our unit was becoming a solidified team, as opposed to various disciplines doing their own thing.

The Occupational Therapists, Physical Therapists and Nurses were acting as a cohesive front to give our patients the total care they needed. The doctor on our unit was also continually praising us and giving us positive feedback on our efforts and treatments.

I feel professionally and personally privileged to have had Harry enter my life. I am lucky to have been able to follow his progress physically and mentally throughout his inpatient stay here at Burke as well as his outpatient and homecare therapy. The changes made in the past nine months have been an amazing journey as well as an inspiration. Harry has made tremendous gains in function, strength and coordination but also in life. He and his wife along with their children represent a unity and bond that goes beyond one's imagination. Dedication and perseverance are two adjectives that come to mind when describing the personalities of Harry and the other survivors that entered our lives here at Burke after 9/11. They are also two adjectives that I have adopted when faced with difficult issues surrounding the scope of Occupational Therapy practice and in my personal life.

The impact of September 11 has been great for many of us as Occupational Therapy practitioners as well as American citizens. It is surprising that we are able to find hope in the face of adversity and something good in the face of tragedy. This past year has presented challenges to therapists and clients at Burke, and we have tackled them with a brave and confident front, all the while dealing with internal struggles and conflicts.

Psychosocial Occupational Therapy Intervention During the 9/11 Tragedy

Mary Squillace, BA, BS/MS, OTR/L

The tragedy of 9/11 helped me to appreciate the need for psychosocial skills and interventions with my physically disabled clients, my friends, my family members, and all of who were affected by this disaster. Returning to work on September 12, the day after, was helpful to some of the people that were mentioned above, but personally, I found it difficult to work. In my roles as an Occupational Therapist, friend and family member, I found myself needing to provide psychosocial direction and/or intervention to many of the people I encountered on a daily basis, but I too needed time to heal myself in order to be effective with others.

The following case presentations are based on true encounters with clients as well as personal acquaintances that were directly affected by the tragic events of September 11. These are individuals whom I interviewed and/or intervened with in order to help them cope with various psychosocial issues that arose from the 9/11 tragedy. These are my nephew, Joe, whose best friend died in the tragedy, and two Muslim families, one from Bangladesh and the other from Afghanistan, whom I worked with as an Occupational Therapist providing home-based early intervention to their infants. I also describe what they taught me, and

[Haworth co-indexing entry note]: "Psychosocial Occupational Therapy Intervention During the 9/11 Tragedy." Squillace, Mary. Co-published simultaneously in *Occupational Therapy in Mental Health* (The Haworth Press, Inc.) Vol. 21, No. 3/4, 2006, pp. 65-73; and: *Healing 9/11: Creative Programming by Occupational Therapists* (ed: Pat Precin) The Haworth Press, Inc., 2006, pp. 65-73. Single or multiple copies of this article are available for a fee from The Haworth Document Delivery Service [1-800- HAWORTH, 9:00 a.m. - 5:00 p.m. (EST). E-mail address: docdelivery@haworthpress.com].

doi:10.1300/J004v21n03_04

how they helped me to cope with my own feelings during this troubled time.

> The ability to identify feelings and need clearly, often a difficulty in the context of the family, can be taught through assertiveness training. A client's ability to respond to the needs of others, sometimes equally problematic, can be taught through cooperative group activities. Also, families need to be given information to understand the deficits of their loved ones. The need to be aware that some behaviors are not willful on the part of the individual, and what strategies they can use to help the individual modulate behaviors. Further, they need to understand how their attitudes and behaviors may contribute to an environment that is not optimal to the individual's performance. (Christiansen & Baum, 1997, p. 329)

CASE PRESENTATION: JOE

Joe and John lived together throughout their college careers and developed a brotherly friendship. John was very close to his family and his death was an enormous loss to them. John also had a girlfriend with whom he was very close. She has yet to recover from his loss.

On September 11, Joe received his first telephone call from a friend who worked nearby, telling him about a fire in the Towers. He recalls his shock at the news, and then as time passed, he grew frightened for himself. Although he was in midtown Manhattan, he felt the fear that thousands of others felt that day. When it occurred to him that John was in one of those buildings, Joe made several unsuccessful attempts to contact him and his family. In the meantime, Joe focused on going to a place where he would feel safe. He lived in downtown Manhattan, so going to his own home was impossible. Later that morning, Joe finally was able to make contact with John's father and felt the latter's fear as they spoke. After a few hours, Joe realized that he had not heard from John. There were many telephone calls from John's friends and family, and Joe finally obtained the fortitude to look for him. That afternoon, Joe and a friend walked downtown in hopes of locating John in the vicinity of the tragedy. Not being able to get too close to the scene, Joe realized the magnitude of this catastrophe and felt he needed to be with the rest of John's close friends. They traveled to Long Island and watched the news in the evening, while they tried to reach John on his cellular telephone. They repeatedly called John's family to see if there was any information on his whereabouts. The next day, there continued to be no word from John. Joe felt the impact of the loss of his good friend. He went to church and cried. John was more like a brother than a friend to Joe.

Joe describes how he felt when he met with John's family, particularly his mother. "She was hysterical. She told me not to touch anything because he was coming home to clean his room. She said not to touch his study notes as she held onto his shirt and would not let go." Joe recalls how his body shook when he initially saw her and how he cried when she hugged him. He had immense feelings of grief and found it difficult to stay at John's place, especially when John's brothers returned home from searching the city shelters. The brothers told their mother that they would find John. Emotions heightened when Joe met with all of their mutual friends that same evening to discuss the possible loss of John. The interaction among the friends was difficult because John was the bond that held the diverse group of acquaintances together. "He was a friend to everyone."

John's girlfriend was and continues to be distraught. She fell into a major depression, quit her job, dropped out of graduate school, and continues to grieve the loss of the love of her life by counting the days he has been gone. They had plans for a future and now those plans were over. John's girlfriend would call Joe many times, especially the first week following the tragedy. "She would call me and cry. She would constantly ask me why this had to happen to John." Joe felt he had to calm her and remain close to her while she grieved. He felt that this was therapeutic for him because the attention he gave to her created a diversion from his own grief.

A memorial was held for John on his birthday. When they found his body, there was a funeral service for him. Joe stated that he felt the familiar overwhelming emotion of grief, and then finally closure. He felt he was able to say goodbye to his friend without any lingering uncertainties of John's whereabouts.

Joe dealt with his grief by speaking to those who were close to him. He states that his girlfriend at the time was of great help to him. She took him to a center that held open meetings discussing the losses of September 11. Joe admitted that he was resistive to attending the meetings, but felt great relief and comfort after only a few sessions. He stated that he spoke with therapists for two hours and experienced an overall sense of reprieve from the harshness of the emotions that were consuming him since the loss of his friend. He developed a fear of speaking with John's parents since John's mother would become very upset when she would see Joe. "She said that every time she would see me it would remind her of John," Joe states. Unintentionally, he created a distance between himself, John's parents, and John's girlfriend. He was concerned that if he were to maintain a relationship with them, it would only be reminiscent of times when John was alive and cause pain between them when they met. After time had passed, Joe began to feel so guilty and hurt that he did not call or contact John's family or girlfriend. He did not want to be reminded of the loss of John or experience the grief and pain he may cause them by contacting them. In October, Joe wrote John's parents a 10-page letter. He wrote about his love for John, their friendship, and how remorseful he was about the distance he created between them. He then made contact with John's parents and apologized. "They were very accepting of my apology. I felt much better once we spoke again." Joe then contacted John's girlfriend and directed her to the appropriate resources for therapy, even though her family was intervening as well.

Joe continues to grieve for his friend. Although he states that he feels he has reached a point of serenity, he becomes teary eyed when he thinks of him. Joe enjoys talking about John with his friends and he often has a smile when topics regarding John transpire. Joe states, "I may not remember my girlfriend's birthday, but I will remember everything that day, every step of the way."

Joe is my nephew. When speaking with him regarding John, I could sense his sorrow and because of our closeness, I could feel his anguish. I told Joe that it would be an excellent consideration to continue with the open discussion sessions or seek other professional help to aid him in his dealings with his remaining grief. I reminded him that it would be appropriate to discuss and be reminiscent of John with his friends and to keep the memory of John active. He should arrange a monthly gathering of John's friends to remind them of the impact and influence John had on all of their lives. I suggested that he remain in contact with John's family, not only for his own satisfaction, but also for John's family who sought out memories of him through Joe.

> Human roles influenced by cultural definition may be limited in the options for role change and reassignment. Patients and their families may assume there is only one way to be a successful man or woman, or a worker, or to fill family membership roles. The considerations of alternative lifestyles and concomitant adult roles may be difficult for the patient and resistive by the family. (Cottrell, 2000, p. 124)

CASE PRESENTATION: THE MUSLIM FAMILIES

The New York City communities are occupied by a variety of ethnicities, religions, cultures, and races. If you are born and raised in one of the boroughs of New York City, you become acclimated to this diversity. Within each community, there may reside a distinct culture. Some of the more common examples of this would be Spanish Harlem, Little Italy, and Chinatown, all in the borough of Manhattan. Certainly, the borough of Queens is a sample community that represents a variety of cultures.

In September of 2001, I was working in Queens with an early intervention home-based program where I was required to go to the homes of infants to offer Occupational Therapy services for varied diagnoses. I did not work on September 11 for obvious reasons, but I did so the following day, and this is what I encountered.

There were two Muslim families on my case load, one family from Bangladesh and the other from Afghanistan, both practicing the Islamic faith. Before September 11, each family had achieved a level of comfort with my presence in their homes consistent with trust and respect for our respective cultures. In fact, we often compared our cultures and discussed their differences.

Upon entering the home of the Afghani family, I felt a dense tension. The mother of the child simply watched me work, without saying a word. At the time, I myself did not feel much like speaking. I was extremely upset and was questioning if it was appropriate to be working so soon, with so little grieving on my part. In place of our usual courteous conversation, she wore a concerned expression and continued not to speak. It appeared as if she were attempting to read my perception of her culture by observing my interactions with her child. There was a definitive uncomfortable silence, so I decided to start the conversation. I started by asking how the child was progressing. Then I demonstrated some techniques that would be advantageous for her to carry over. She agreed to do so. When our eyes met, it was obvious that we were experiencing the same sorrow and pain. She began immediately explaining that what had occurred the day before was not demonstrative of the Muslim's beliefs within the Islamic faith. She agreed that the events were extremely horrific and she mentioned that she prayed for the healing of the suffering of the American people. She began to describe to me the meaning of the Islamic faith. How it is based on peaceful thoughts and ideas and that what had happened was evil. I listened to her explain how grateful she and her family were to have an opportunity to live in the United States. She presented with a nervous demeanor when we spoke, especially in regard to the individuals who participated in the terror acts. At that time, I was still very sensitive to the catastrophe and did not expect her explanations. We then spoke in detail about what had happened. The conversation was an in-depth discussion, involving the ignorance of people. She was concerned regarding how others would perceive her if she were to appear in her community in her burka and was fearful to go outdoors. She wore a complete burka with the nekab, the part that covers the eyes of its wearer. I mentioned that this day it would not be a good idea walk outside in her burka. I told her that people would see only what she was wearing and react with ignorance, disrespect, and anger. She mentioned that her husband had called to tell her to remain inside and that he will pick up the groceries upon his return home from work.

Within a few weeks, our relationship returned to a more comfortable level. Our interaction was one of a newfound level of respect for our cultures. Primarily, our conversations included topics involving her son and his future progress. As time passed, she became less fearful of going outdoors, and I learned a tremendous amount regarding her culture.

> Some environmental attributes interact with human capabilities to enable performance, while others present barriers to an individual's attempts at meaningful interactions with his or her surroundings. (Christiansen & Baum, 1997, p. 338)

Within another home a similar situation occurred. Although the mother of this child and I had already established a friendly relationship, we found ourselves searching for answers to perplexing questions about our faiths. When I arrived at her home, her initial reaction to my presence was an apologetic one for what she felt was a gross example of inhumanity. She expressed how remorseful she felt about the entire situation. She stated, "This is not what we practice. It is very unfortunate that this is the only example of the Islamic faith Americans may see, and we are totally opposite of that." She also had the same concerns regarding her appearance within the community. She, too, wore a burka. The difference is that she wears a hijab, which is a handkerchief covering her head instead of the full head and face covering. There was much apprehension to go outdoors, but her desire to do so surmounted that anxiety. She stated, "I suddenly feel trapped and do not want to be a prisoner within my home." She then asked if I would walk with her to the store because she felt that she would be less likely to encounter any overt prejudices or harm than if she went by herself. Admittedly, I felt slightly nervous with this request. This neighborhood was not considered one of the safest communities in Queens and, besides fear, there was a fresh sense of anger and frustration throughout New York. I was honest with her regarding my apprehension, and I agreed to go if it would relieve her anxiety, but suggested we should remain indoors for the next few days before attempting that mission. We agreed that because she was a more liberated Muslim, she would wear slacks with a casual shirt and a hijab.

Two days later, all was solemn within the community, but there continued to be an intense feeling of sadness. As we walked toward a small local fruit and vegetable stand, there was a sense that a constant eye was upon us. My client's mother made mention of this feeling, and I reassured her that this sense is exaggerated by our already present anxiety. We were silent for some time as we scanned the surroundings. Then she said nervously, "This is it; they are going to kill me." I assured her, as she already knew, that was not going to happen. I decided to distract her to help her regain her security within her environment by discussing her son's accomplishments and goals. This technique worked and we slowly regained a comfortable sense of security within our surroundings and our selves.

> Occupational therapy is grounded in principles and values that honor the rights and potential of every client, whether that client is a corporation, community, group, or an individual. These principles are reflected in every thoughtful interaction between therapist and client. At its best, occupational therapy is an apparently simple process that helps clients make order and meaning out of complex and challenging situations. This deceptively simple process is, in fact, multidimensional, collaborative, and creative. It enables clients to envision their futures to the extent that they are willing to work toward them. This means that the worked-for future must have meaning and value to the individual clients. (Law, 1998, p. 67)

These subject presentations are only three of the many interactions that I have encountered during the 9/11 tragedy. The similarity of these incidences is that emotional suffering occurred in each case entirely because of one tragedy.

Time has passed and it appears as though society has presently returned to a homeostasis. Although our anxieties considering a possible new tragedy or disaster are ever present, we continue to function out of necessity for monetary and emotional purposes.

To some, returning to the work force was a break from the reality of the events of 9/11. "Work helps me to keep my mind off of the loss of John," Joe told me. He returned to work soon after the loss of his friend. "I started work the Monday after 9/11. I was making myself crazy by constantly wondering and worrying about John. So, I decided to go to work because I had to. I am busy at work and I knew my mind would be occupied with my work and not John. Do not get me wrong, I did think of him often, but I did not have time to dwell on it. Working helped me to move on."

Soon after the tragedy, the employment rates plummeted and layoffs were widespread. As a result, both of the Muslim families that were mentioned suffered from these layoffs. Both of the husbands had lost their jobs approximately three to four months after September 11. One of the men, who had earned a doctoral degree in electrical engineering, was forced to move his family into the basement of a friend's house until he can find employment again. But he faces a more serious problem. He was working in the United States on a sponsorship from his job and he is awaiting the arrival of his green card in order to stay in the country. "I understand that I may have to go back to 'my country' [Afghanistan] if I do not find another sponsor that will employ me. We cannot continue to live in someone else's home." His wife mentioned to me that she feels he is experiencing a serious depression. The only advice that I could offer her was for her to help him search the Internet for sponsorships while they await the green card. I was truly at a loss for words for her.

There comes a time when, we, the health care professionals, need to capture time to restore our own bearings and attempt to mend our own broken spirit. The repeated broaching of the same topic by our clients has an ability to sneak up on us, especially with a subject of such extreme sensitive content that can arouse emotions that appear to be universal.

People who choose to work within the health care field have extraordinary personalities. I think that it is a collective opinion that the motivating factor of being an Occupational Therapist is not solely for monetary purposes, but more so for an unselfish desire or need to help others. We enter into the field of Occupational Therapy aware that we are dedicating our lives to assisting others in need of rehabilitation. And yet, the reality is that it is more than just a physical rehabilitative service that we offer. With that in mind, we are conscious of the situation in which we place ourselves. On some level we are expected to behave in a manner that is calming to others, have the answers to many troubles, and to be a resource of information that will help in regaining our client's premorbid lives. Therefore, we have the ability to appropriately alter our disposition pertaining to each individual case while maintaining the professionalism we are trained to demonstrate.

Working so soon after this tragic event was difficult for myself. Everyday I was confronted with other people's heartaches and concerns, and everyday I thought that I was placed in a position to console. My desire to offer sentiments was present, but I was not positive that it would be possible to do so without imposing my opinion or my own emotional instability regarding the topic. I was sensitive to the fact that these clients were searching for answers and required a suitable response. With each interaction, there was an uncertainty as to whether my responses or suggestions were correct. After all, how could I possibly propose ideas to others when I felt the implications of my suggestions might be inapt? Simply, I felt helpless at times and it would be an undesirable act to demonstrate my weaknesses at their time of need. For the most part, the only effective resolution was to simply listen to my clients.

Although working very soon after the event may have been difficult for me, it also helped me to gain the strength that I needed to face another day. My clients gave me that strength. In working with such a diverse population, with an assortment of problems, I learned that everyone suffers the same during such tragic times. This event enabled me to be appreciative of a skill that allows others to confide in me with an exceptional degree of trust and confidence.

REFERENCES

Christiansen, C. & Baum, C. (1997). *Occupational therapy: Enabling function and well-being* (2nd ed.). Thorofare, NJ: Slack Incorporated, pp. 329 & 338.

Cottrell, R. & Fleming, P. (2000). *Proactive approaches in psychosocial occupational therapy*. Thorofare, NJ: Slack Incorporated, p. 124.

Law, M. (1998). *Client-centered occupational therapy*. Thorofare, NJ: Slack Incorporated, p. 67.

PHOTO 1. Boy Drawing the Twin Towers with Chalk on a New York City Street. A Heart Is Emerging from the Tower.

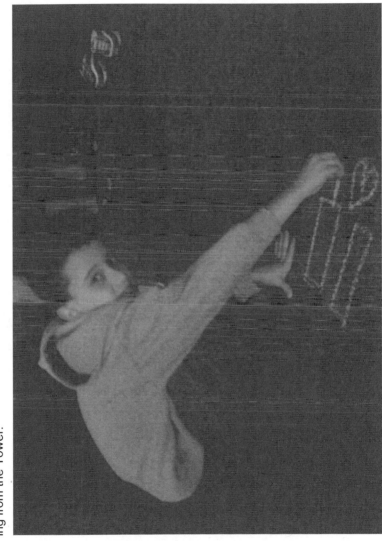

Moving to New York City:
Helping 9/11 Children

Christina Hughes, MS, OTR/L

LEAVING THE WOODS OF CHAPEL HILL

I could not sleep.

It was 2:00 on the morning of September 11, 2001. I found myself wide-awake, staring at the ceiling. This was highly unusual for me. I usually slept through the night undisturbed. I had awakened with a disturbing feeling of dread. The cat was sleeping peacefully in her usual spot at the edge of the bed, giving me some assurance that the danger existed only in my mind. Restless, I finally got up and walked out onto the back porch. The moon shone through the trees and an occasional owl hooted but all else was quiet in the woods of Chapel Hill, North Carolina.

Why such a feeling of dread? Maybe it is because of the move.

I was moving to New York City shortly, but the timing was contingent upon receiving my Occupational Therapy license. For some reason, I was eager to get to New York but equally reluctant to leave my home in the woods of Chapel Hill.

Moving to Queens, New York, with my best friend Tim, an international flight attendant for United States Airways, would be an experience! Our sublet apartment, located right on the East River, had a

[Haworth co-indexing entry note]: "Moving to New York City: Helping 9/11 Children." Hughes, Christina. Co-published simultaneously in *Occupational Therapy in Mental Health* (The Haworth Press, Inc.) Vol. 21, No. 3/4, 2006, pp. 77-94; and: *Healing 9/11: Creative Programming by Occupational Therapists* (ed: Pat Precin) The Haworth Press, Inc., 2006, pp. 77-94. Single or multiple copies of this article are available for a fee from The Haworth Document Delivery Service [1-800- HAWORTH, 9:00 a.m. - 5:00 p.m. (EST). E-mail address: docdelivery@haworthpress.com].

Available online at http://www.haworthpress.com/web/OTMH
doi:10.1300/J004v21n03_05

panoramic view of Manhattan. I had no job in New York, no savings, and no license. These facts made me nervous, but they did not explain the dread.

I continued to sit on the back porch thinking about the move. Several hours passed before it was finally possible for me to fall asleep. The next morning, waking about 10:00 and still feeling weird, I began to wonder if this was an anxiety attack. I had certainly never felt like this before. The day's agenda included working per diem at a nursing home in Durham. I was just about to leave when the phone rang. My friend Donald was on the line, and he sounded shaky.

"Christina, have you heard the news?" his voice cracking as he asked. My heart began to beat hard. Because I did not own a television or radio, my friends frequently called when a major news story was developing.

"Two planes took out both towers of the World Trade Center, a third hit the Pentagon, and a fourth crashed outside of Pittsburgh."

That explained the dread.

Working at the nursing home that day was difficult. Staff spoke of the tragedy and many wondered aloud what they could do. I called the Office of Professions in Albany, hoping that my license had been approved. Within the next few days, a sense of normalcy returned to the nursing home, at least on the surface. But for me, everything had changed. I was more determined than ever to get to New York.

On September 13, 2001, my New York State Occupational Therapy license was approved. It was my 33rd birthday a day later. To me, that license was the best gift I could have received. Most people did not understand my happiness; even I could not explain it fully at the time.

Tim was safe but stuck in Amsterdam. He had been working during September 11 and could not get back to the United States until planes started flying again. He called me from Philadelphia, where he was based, as soon as he got back into the country. We asked each other the same question,

"Are you still planning on moving?"

We both had the same answer, a resounding, "Yes."

I packed the car, put my cat in the passenger's seat, and left North Carolina. After picking up Tim in Philadelphia on September 18, we drove up to the toll booth at the George Washington Bridge ready to cross the Hudson River and enter New York. There was virtually no traffic except for us and a few scattered cars. I had never seen the city so desolate at rush hour; it was eerie.

UNION SQUARE AND THE WORLD TRADE CENTER

Tim and I arrived at our apartment, dropped our suitcases, and walked to the park a block away where we could gaze across the East River and behold all of Manhattan. The month before we could look south and see the Twin Towers. Now they were gone. Huge clouds of billowing smoke streamed upward into the sky where the World Trade Center once stood (Photo 2). It was the first time the magnitude of the event struck me. We continued to stare at lower Manhattan as we called friends and family to let them know we had arrived safely.

Later that evening, Tim and I went to Union Square, a memorial site for all those who were missing or dead. There were posters of missing people everywhere (Photo 3), in subway stations, on telephone poles, and throughout Union Square. Every inch of the park was covered with candles of various shapes and sizes (Photo 4). People shuffled around in disbelief. Some played songs on their guitars. Others volunteered to keep the candles burning. Most just congregated. As United States President George Walker Bush cried out for justice, the people at Union Square prayed for peace. There was a collective presence in the park I had never felt before. In the face of tragedy, I felt the unexpected emotion of joy as I heard the resounding cry for peace. My body tingled; my eyes stung with tears.

Walking through Union Square, I came across a young woman whose behavior captured my interest. Most people were moving from place to place, talking quietly, crying, or playing music (Photos 5 and 6). This woman did none of those things. She simply sat on the ground and held out her burning candle towards the thousands of others that were lit. Her eyes were open. She said nothing. In the face of so much movement and emotion, she seemingly did the impossible. She sat perfectly still.

The next morning I took the subway and headed downtown to the site where the Twin Towers once stood. I had stayed at the Marriott World Trade Center in 1996 and still had a hard time believing it was gone. The first thing to hit me was the smell. It was biting, raw, and acrid. People were walking around wearing white masks. It was raining and windy. I clung to my umbrella while covering my nose with my shirtsleeve hoping to filter some of the odor.

The police and National Guard were everywhere. There were a few people with video cameras, but the crowds had yet to come out in full force. It was easy to get within a half block of the site and to look, except there was nothing to see but rubble. Both structures were completely

PHOTO 2. Observers in New Jersey Are Watching a Smoldering Manhattan Across the Hudson River.

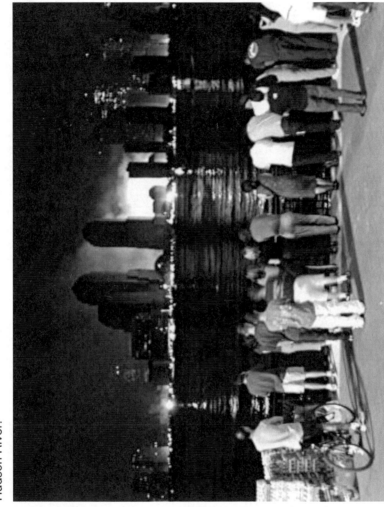

PHOTO 3. Poster of Missing People.

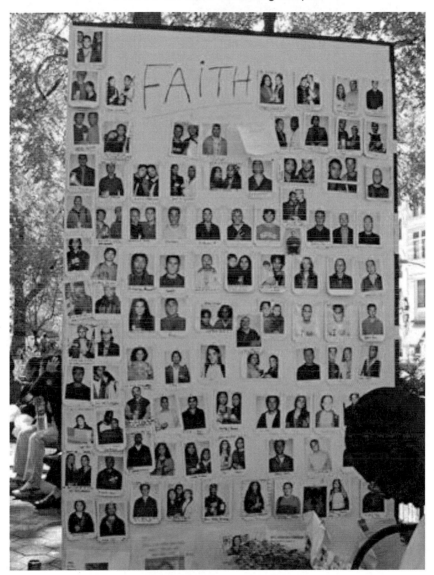

Photo by Donna Brennan. Used by permission.

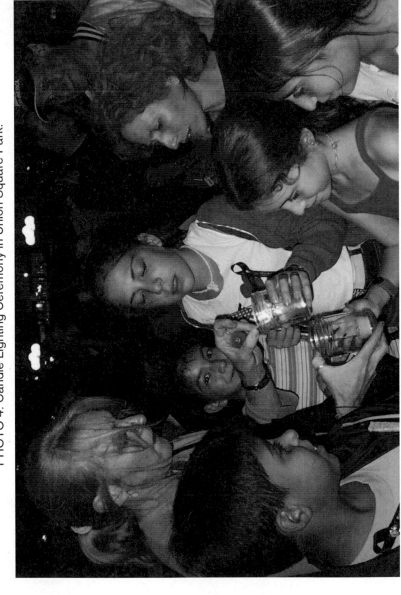

PHOTO 4. Candle Lighting Ceremony in Union Square Park.

Photo by Pat Precin. Used by permission.

PHOTO 5. Drumming for Freedom in Union Square Park.

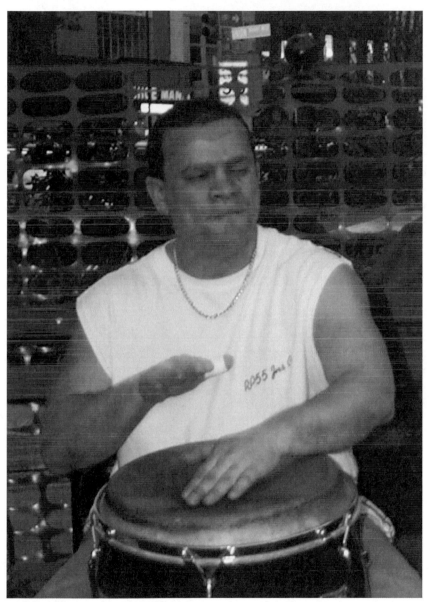

Photo by Pat Precin. Used by permission.

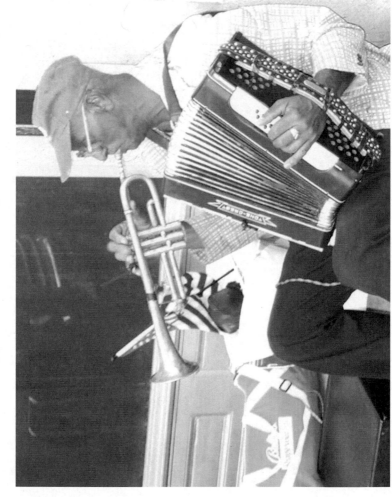

leveled. There was one small part left of one of the towers that consisted of burnt-out steel girders (Photo 7). It was the snapshot that all the magazines and newspapers featured.

I did not stay that long. There was nothing to see. I did not feel sad. I felt empty. It was as if thousands of people had packed up and moved away. But that was not true. I never went back to the site. I never felt the need to do so. By contrast, Union Square became an area that I visited frequently.

BEDFORD-STUYVESANT IS NOT PARK SLOPE

I needed to start working right away since all of my meager assets had been spent on apartment expenses. In speaking with a Manhattan contract company, I felt certain I could begin working with them. They were reputable and honest. A meeting was arranged with Tricia, my main contact at this agency, to discuss available pediatric opportunities. Despite my practical needs, though, instinct told me that this was not quite the right placement. Attempting to reassure myself that I wanted to work in Manhattan and that this was a good contract company did nothing to allay my uneasiness. At the meeting's conclusion I thanked Tricia and said I would be in touch. Why had I trusted this feeling? Rent was coming due and I had nothing in the bank! Although there was a demand for Occupational Therapists in New York City, I knew it might take some time to find the right position.

I went home and started faxing out resumes. A couple who lived on the 27th floor of my building befriended me and let me use their fax machine. The gentleman was a professor and his wife worked at the United Nations. Both were Muslims. They seemed surprised and happy that I was moving to New York immediately following September 11. We discussed recent events as I faxed resume after resume. They asked me about Occupational Therapy, what it was, and what I did. They were very kind and our interaction seemed reassuring to all of us. For them, to know that someone would treat them no differently than before the 9/11 attacks, and for me to start meeting people in a city where I knew no one except for my friend Tim.

Almost immediately, I received a call from a contract company that had several schools needing an Occupational Therapist in the Park Slope section of Brooklyn. I was excited. Park Slope was a nice area. At this point, I was happy there were still positions left in desirable schools since it was almost October.

PHOTO 7. A Small Part of a Tower Remains.

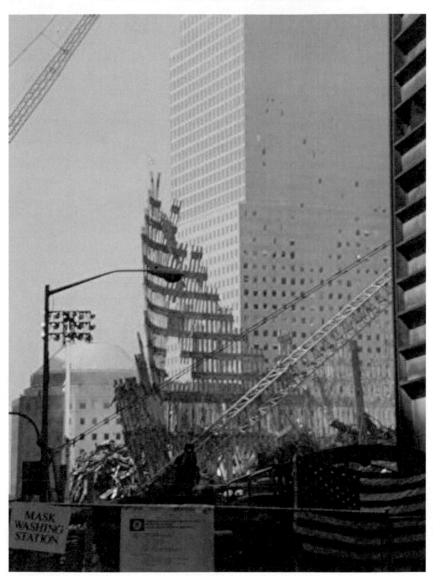

Photo by Donna Brennan. Used by permission.

I took the subway downtown to meet the special education coordinators of four potential schools. Exiting the subway, however, I found myself in Bedford Stuyvesant, not Park Slope. I looked around at the run-down storefronts and abandoned houses. Young people were hanging out on the corners listening to rap music that was blasting from state-of-the-art stereo systems in brand new sport utility vehicles. I knew Bedford Stuyvesant had the reputation for being a tough area. The contract company knew that too. So they renamed it Park Slope.

Walking through the neighborhood, I had some difficulty finding my first school so I asked a woman on the street. She pointed diagonally over a couple of blocks.

"It is that school that looks like it is closed because it has bars on all the windows."

All I could see were high-rise housing projects. Nevertheless, I began walking in that direction. Sure enough, a school matching the woman's description emerged after a few minutes.

I trudged up to the fifth floor to meet Ms. Heather Hunte, the special education coordinator. A short woman in her forties, she had long dark hair and wore glasses and a business suit. Ms. Hunte performed three different tasks as she answered my questions in rapid-fire succession. There were two children in her office quietly working on different activities. Ms. Hunte explained that there was a mixture of children receiving Occupational Therapy. Some were in regular education while others were in self-contained classrooms. If a child was in a regular education classroom, he or she was cognitively functioning at grade level. A self-contained classroom placement indicated the child either needed more time to complete age appropriate academics or was not able to do grade level work. Many students had problems with behavior and several were diagnosed with attention deficit disorder. Several of the children had challenging home lives and either lived with one parent or relatives.

As we finished talking, I sat there for a minute and stared out the window unsure if I should work at this school. There was a tape playing in the background; and, as if she could read my mind, Ms. Hunte turned up that stereo and began to sing in the strongest, most beautiful voice. It brought tears to my eyes, and I nonchalantly tried to wipe them away. I had not planned on an emotional interview. I told Ms. Hunte I needed to think about working at the school, but would be in touch with her by the next day.

I shook my head in wonderment over this unanticipated development. I had lived and worked in an inner city environment for several years previously but thought those days were over. I had moved to New York to work in Manhattan, not Brooklyn. As I walked to the G train on Nostrand Avenue, I asked out loud, "Here?"

"Here!" an inner voice answered.

I started work at Ms. Hunte's school the next day.

THE CHILDREN

By the beginning of October, I was the Occupational Therapist in two Bedford-Stuyvesant elementary schools. In addition, I was treating one preschool home-care client in an affluent section of Manhattan on the Upper East Side. Though the areas were polar opposites in some ways, I learned a great deal working in these diverse and sometimes divergent sections of New York.

On the first day of work, I came to Ms. Hunte's office armed with my laptop and photocopy paper. While waiting for her to show me the children's files, I gazed out the fifth floor office window at a view of lower Manhattan–something I had not noticed on my previous visit. The school psychologist observed me looking off into the distance.

"Ms. Hunte and I used to have a view of the World Trade Center," he stated matter-of-factly, "but no more."

I nodded, beginning to realize that this school was the reason I was here in New York.

"All the children on the North side saw the planes hit." The psychologist gestured toward the part of the school building where we were standing. I wondered what impact this event had on the children. I was about to find out in subsequent treatment sessions.

My first project with the students involved getting them to think about what they wanted to be when they grew up. Some had difficulty choosing just one occupation so the children could write about as many careers as they wished. Once they had decided, the students wrote out a rough draft on a lined piece of paper which we then corrected for spelling and grammatical errors. Students copied their rough draft onto black lined paper using different colored gel pens. Each child then drew a picture to accompany their writing either freehand or using stencils. Most of the children had never used gel pens or stencils before. It took them several sessions to complete this project and all of them appeared to enjoy expressing themselves in this manner.

Several students wanted to be firemen or policemen. They drew pictures of people helping others out of the World Trade Center. They drew the Twin Towers as well. I noticed that the children who decided on these professions did so almost instantaneously. Occupational Therapy was giving them a medium not only to express their future occupations but also to discuss the World Trade Center in terms that they could understand. The children were more likely to speak about the collapse of the Twin Towers while they were doing an activity. Talk alone did not appear as effective.

In my previous experience working with inner city students, children usually picked careers such as rappers, basketball players, football players, and wrestlers. When I would ask why they chose these particular occupations, they generally had two reasons: (1) they could make a lot of money, and (2) these jobs were considered to be fun rather than work.

This was the first time I had observed an unprecedented number of students choosing careers that were realistic; the children were aware that police and firemen did not make a lot of money and these professions were indeed very hard work. I could only surmise that the shift in career choices was a positive effect born out of the tragedy of the World Trade Center.

For the first few months, my students built Twin Towers out of everything available to them, including clay and various types of blocks. When these sessions occurred, they followed a typical pattern. A child would build the World Trade Center, then construct a plane to knock the towers down.

Children frequently asked questions without prompting, such as: "What should happen to the terrorists who were involved in this event?"

This was the number one question by far. Some students believed anyone involved should be imprisoned for life while others thought terrorists should be executed for killing so many people. While the children expressed their beliefs, I remained neutral and assisted them with the reasoning that brought them to these conclusions. This type of treatment session gave the children the opportunity to get to know me while expressing their feelings on a historical event that had happened in their city.

Throughout the year, many events involving the World Trade Center disaster touched my heart. One such event involved the many support banners sent to this school from people throughout the United States. One December day, I walked into a second grade classroom where they had just received a banner from California. I happened to be carrying my portable blow-up Earth that doubled as a globe. It looked very much like a beach ball. When the teacher saw the Earth, her eyes lit up.

"Can I see that for a second?" she asked.

I tossed her the Earth and she showed the second grade class where California was in relation to New York. It was one of the most spontaneous educable moments I can remember involving the World Trade Center.

The banners and posters gave me the opportunity to show students the states and cities where they came from, as the teacher above had done. This is especially important for children in the inner city because most do not frequently travel outside their immediate neighborhoods. As a result, geography can often be confusing to them because they have a more localized reference point.

I had a map of the United States that was a puzzle with the shape of each state representing one piece. Every time I noticed a new banner or poster, the student and I would find that state and see where it was in relation to New York. We would then assemble all the states in between. For example, when a banner was sent from Tennessee, the student would identify which state was Tennessee, which state was New York, and then use the puzzle box as a guide and piece together all the states North of Tennessee and South of New York. The children were more likely to remember a state if they had a personal connection to it. They would recall Tennessee because that is where the banner originated. As we pieced together the puzzle, they would usually recognize places like Pennsylvania and New Jersey because they had been there before. This excited them as they began to understand where states that had sent us banners and places they had traveled to were in relation to where they lived.

There were many teachable moments like this. I felt fortunate because whenever the World Trade Center came up in a treatment session, I was able to devote time to the topic and construct an activity around the discussion. The teachers did not have this flexibility. A few days immediately following the tragedy had been devoted to writing and talking about the event; but, ultimately, there was a curriculum to follow. Occupational Therapy was a place where the children could express the various emotions they felt through educational meaningful activities.

My second school was located in the same neighborhood. Most of the students on my caseload were in self-contained classrooms with approximately a third to half of my caseload diagnosed with Down's Syndrome. The younger children I serviced at this school did not understand what had happened to the World Trade Center. The older ones understood the events, but not necessarily the impact on people's lives.

In one particular treatment session, an 11-year-old child diagnosed with mental retardation built the World Trade Center out of blocks then knocked it down with a pencil that was a pretend plane. He proceeded to laugh heartily. When I asked him what was funny, he explained that he thought the planes crashing into the buildings were funny. He had seen this numerous times on television. This student then mentioned several television shows where explosions and crashes happened routinely.

I found his reaction very disturbing but fought hard to put my personal feelings aside. Although this session made me angry, I did not want to reprimand this student. It was evident that he was likening the World Trade Center to a television show. He did not appear able to distinguish fantasy from reality in this situation. Using language and descriptions he could understand, I explained why the events of the World Trade Center were different than watching a television show, keeping my description short and concise. I did not dwell on the disaster itself but instead sought to explain the difference between reality and make-believe.

This child never laughed again about the World Trade Center as far as I know–not because he fully distinguished the event from a television show, but because he saw the reaction his laughter provoked.

One other student had the same reaction. He was also an 11-year-old diagnosed with mental retardation in the same self-contained classroom. I wondered if either child remotely understood the magnitude of the events that had taken place on September 11. My question was answered in mid-June 2002, the day when the last steel girder (Photo 8) was cleared away from the World Trade Center site. The teacher of these two children had brought in a television so her class could watch the ceremony. All 12 students, including the two boys, watched the ceremony with a reverence I had never witnessed before. Frequently, they were very loud, had short attention spans, and were unable to remain in their desks for any length of time. But on that day, all the children were seated in silence with rapt attention, watching the screen. I had not seen anything like it all year. I was in awe that the students were capable of such reverence. Perhaps these students did not see the World Trade Center disaster the way the rest of the world did, but they sensed it in their own way. They knew it was important.

Throughout the school year, I rode the subway twice a week traveling uptown to the Upper East Side in Manhattan to work with a three and a half year old named Kevin with general developmental delay. This was his first year in private preschool. His brother, Joshua (both boy's names have been changed to protect their identity), was five years old and though I did not service him, Joshua was present for the majority of treatment sessions. He attended a private kindergarten. I worked at the

PHOTO 8. The Final Steel Girders at the World Trade Center Site.

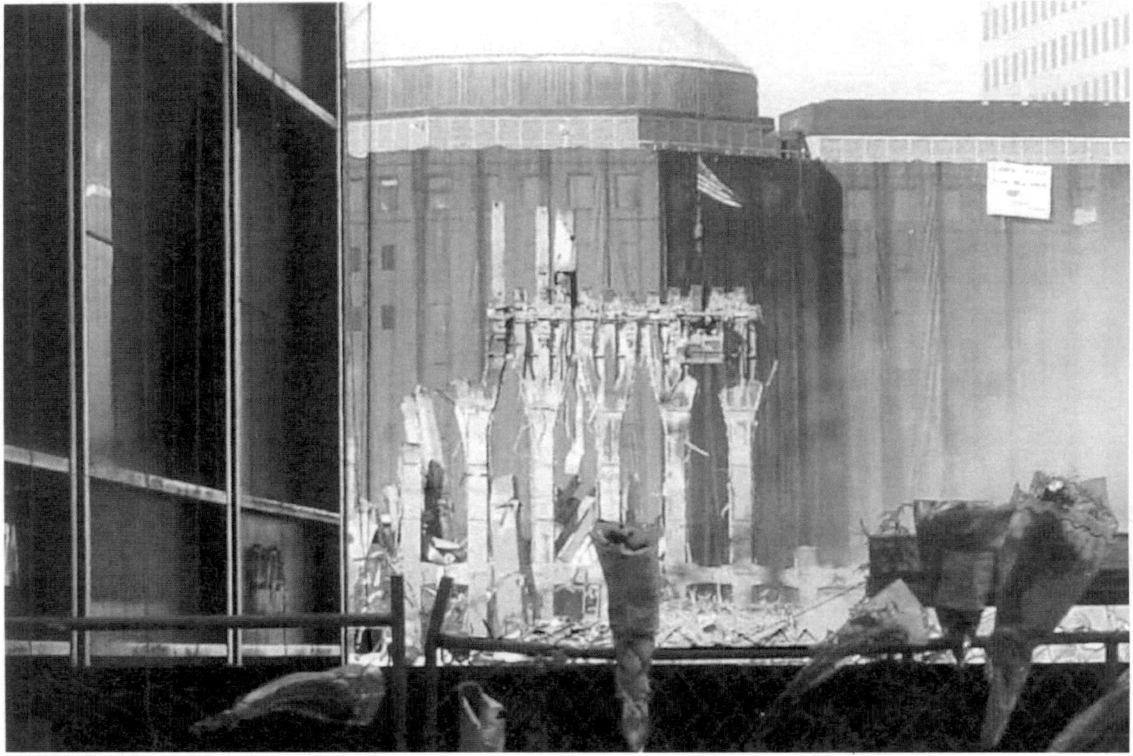

Photo by Donna Brennan. Used by permission.

home for a substantial period of time during each treatment session. Joshua, in particular, was extremely articulate and was well versed on a variety of subjects.

The boys never mentioned the World Trade Center disaster during the eight months I worked with them.

Kevin and Joshua's parents appeared to be able to shield them from the impact. They were not allowed to watch television or play video games during the week. The boys did not see the planes hit the Twin Towers again and again and again. (By contrast, many of the children I serviced in Bedford Stuyvesant watched television or played video games the majority of the time they were at home. In fact, many fell asleep in front of the television in the early morning hours and as a result could not pay attention in class.)

The family was also able to travel outside of the city and did so frequently. The boys' grandfather had a home on Long Island that Joshua referred to as their "weekend house." In addition, the family visited various vacation spots such as Florida and California when the boys were off from school. Unlike the children in Bedford Stuyvesant, Kevin and Joshua knew geography extremely well for their ages.

I believe that the family's ability to travel and established parental controls enabled the parents to minimize the events the World Trade Center disaster had on their children's lives. The young age of the children may have also contributed to their non-reaction, although I perceive this as a lesser factor.

It is likely that the parents did discuss the World Trade Center disaster with their sons when it first occurred, but it is unknown to me how either boy felt about the Twin Towers collapsing. No pictures were ever drawn, no towers were ever constructed, and no words were ever spoken about this event.

THE RESILIENCE OF NEW YORKERS

Early October 2001 found me at Apple Bank in Union Square opening a business account. The customer service representative who assisted me asked about my business and what I did. I gave her a brief description of Occupational Therapy and why I had moved to New York at this particular time. In return, she volunteered some information about herself.

"I have lived in Lower Manhattan all my life–right off Canal Street and I tell you I have never seen the city like this. No one knows what is going to happen next. But people . . . they are talking to each other like never before. I guess disaster makes you want to help each other out. It is rare you get to see that here."

When she finished opening my account, she reached across her desk and shook my hand,

"Welcome. You are a New Yorker now."

Tears stung my eyes and I truly realized why I had moved. There is nothing more uplifting than the resilience of New Yorkers. To be among them this past year watching them rebuild their city was an honor. I had so many people ask me, "Why would you want to move there during such a disastrous time?"

My response was always the same, "Because I had the chance to see the city at its best."

As this chapter details, everyone dealt with the World Trade Center disaster differently. Children and adults alike did the best they could and then they moved on. Perhaps that is the most important part of the story. The collapse of the Twin Towers was a fact of life for everyone. But it did not stop New Yorkers from going forward with their lives, my students included. As an Occupational Therapist, I was so very privileged to play a small part in the recovery effort. And as a result, something I never anticipated happened.

I fell in love with the people of New York City.

Coping with September 11th:
An Occupational Therapist Faculty
Member's Perspective

Mary Beth Early, MS, OTR/L

DAY ONE–BEARING WITNESS

For September, the weather was both typical and gorgeous, unusually hot, sunny, and brilliantly filled with possibilities. A clear blue sky stretched above the buildings all around, silhouetting the red brick and brownstone homes and green leaves and subtle bark of trees. Since I had no classes scheduled for Tuesday, the day was my own. On my way to the swimming pool at the Brooklyn YWCA at 6:30 a.m., I stopped at a local public school to vote in the primary election, but the voting booths were not set up. Birdsong and the occasional car horn were pleasant normal sounds as I got my son off to school, and went back to vote.

Typically, on Tuesday mornings, it is my habit to travel by subway to Manhattan for a yoga class. But I decided instead to visit a Walgreen's on Third and Atlantic Avenues in Brooklyn, near my home, to pick up some items that might make my life easier in returning to teaching after major reconstructive hand surgery. Approaching Atlantic Avenue at about 8:45, I heard and saw a fender-bender accident–not unusual on a busy six-lane conduit at rush hour. About 15 minutes later as I was paying for my items the honking and other rush hour noises felt different.

[Haworth co-indexing entry note]: "Coping with September 11th: An Occupational Therapist Faculty Member's Perspective." Early, Mary Beth. Co-published simultaneously in *Occupational Therapy in Mental Health* (The Haworth Press, Inc.) Vol. 21, No. 3/4, 2006, pp. 95-105; and: *Healing 9/11: Creative Programming by Occupational Therapists* (ed: Pat Precin) The Haworth Press, Inc., 2006, pp. 95-105. Single or multiple copies of this article are available for a fee from The Haworth Document Delivery Service [1-800-HAWORTH, 9:00 a.m. - 5:00 p.m. (EST). E-mail address: docdelivery@haworthpress.com].

Available online at http://www.haworthpress.com/web/OTMH
doi:10.1300/J004v21n03_06

The cashier said that a plane had flown into the World Trade Center. I moved toward the exit doors, looking up to see smoke pouring from the north tower, about a mile or a mile and a half away. It was 9:01 a.m.

With my eyes on the burning tower, I walked along Atlantic toward home, observing people standing in small groups and singly, some with hands over their mouths, gazing in the same direction. Walking down the block, I watched as the second tower exploded. What did I feel? Horror, fear, grief, astonishment, and confusion. . . I knew intuitively that this was an act of terrorism or war. Concerns about biological and chemical agents were in my mind, as was the fear of future attacks.

Arriving home, I phoned my parents in California, to let them know that I was all right and not to worry. My son was at a middle school in Brooklyn (a mile further from the twin towers), and my husband was teaching at a high school on the East Side of lower Manhattan, within walking distance of the World Trade Center. I worried about both of them, and decided to stay near the phone. I heard from neither until the school day ended. They were fine.

For most of the first two hours after the second plane hit, I stayed indoors, close to the telephone, hooked up to the Internet via dial-up and America Online, sending IMs (instant messages) back and forth to one of my sisters in New Jersey. Each tower fell with a muted and prolonged terrible rumble that could be felt and heard in my living room. (We had experienced a house collapse following a gas explosion two blocks away the previous summer and it sounded the same, just farther away, bigger, and terribly prolonged.)

During the day, I tried to remain calm and constructive. I phoned the college, made decisions about classes for the occupational therapy assistant program (of which I was acting director at the time), spoke with faculty members, and thought about what I could do that would be helpful. I stood outside with the cordless phone as evacuees covered with ash walked down my quiet residential tree-lined street of 19th century brick and brownstone row houses. Most did not speak, staring ahead fixedly or with downcast eyes. One man asked to use my phone, which by then was no longer working.

Later, I went upstairs and did some quiet restorative yoga, a calming forward-bending sequence. As smoke began to fill the air in our part of Brooklyn, I closed the windows and turned on the air conditioners. I went outside to the back garden and filled the bird feeders, feeling as one with the twittering confusion and anxiety of the finches and sparrows.

Many hours later, by prior arrangement, my son walked home with a police detective (mother of my son's friend) along with several other boys. Fine dust was in his hair and on his backpack and clothing. He took a shower and I washed everything he wore or brought home. My husband arrived in the late afternoon, carrying groceries and seeming oblivious to our concern for him (demonstrating his style of coping through cooking, eating and exercising). We were all so relieved to be together, and despite the day's tragedy, my husband and son found solace in the news that the public schools would be closed for the foreseeable future.

We learned, however, that a long-time acquaintance (of almost 30 years) was missing, having been at work at Marsh Incorporated that morning. She had been the first girlfriend of my husband's best friend, and we had seen her many times over the years. On that day, we were all thinking of her as missing and only gradually understood that this would mean missing forever.

RETURNING TO WORK–LIFE AT THE COLLEGE

Although much of New York City was shut down the following day, Wednesday September 12, and most city workers were told to stay home, the City University of New York was open. Classes at LaGuardia Community College would be held. Faculty was notified to be present. Awaking early (if I slept at all) I drove through eerily deserted streets, past police blockades of the major bridges and the 911 command center, and was redirected by police several times before I found my way to work.

LaGuardia Community College is unusual in several aspects. It is very large (11,000 students in the year 2001) and is located in Queens, a populous and diverse borough to the east of Manhattan. LaGuardia's current slogan is "the world's community college," with over 1100 foreign students representing 108 countries enrolled during the 2001-02 school year. An additional 4,300 enrolled students immigrated to the United States from their native countries. Thus, almost half of enrolled students were born outside the United States.

The 14 students enrolled in Occupational Therapy Skills and Functional Activities 1 included representatives from the following countries: Dominican Republic, Grenada, Guyana, Haiti, India, Iran, the Philippines, Poland, and Uzbekistan. Two students were Muslim, several others Roman Catholic. Thirteen of the students were female. All fourteen students were present for their first class on Monday, September 10. Eight arrived for class on Wednesday, September 12. The syllabus listed the following topics for that day: Overview of Occupational Therapy Evaluation Process and Role of the Occupational Therapy Assistant; Introduction to Interviewing and Clinical Observation Skills; Methods of Data Collection and Intervention; and Note Writing (continuation of exercise from Monday's class). I asked the students if they would like to go with Plan A (the syllabus topics) or Plan B (something to help us all process what had happened and was happening). We agreed to go with Plan B.

Circle Sharing

We first gathered in a circle, seated in armless classroom chairs. I invited the students to share their experiences. One student spoke of watching from her high-rise building through binoculars, and seeing things falling from the towers, and then perceiving suddenly that those were not pieces of paper or furniture, but people jumping. She shook and sobbed as she described this. The student sitting next to her reached for and held her hand. Another tearfully told of a family member who was missing. Most of the others said only a few words and one chose very deliberately to remain silent.

I explained to the group that not talking was all right, and that if they changed their minds I would be available to listen, either here in the group or later in my office privately. I asked if anyone had anything further to share, waited a minute or two, and then asked if they wanted to attempt a relaxation exercise. With the group's agreement, we moved on to the second activity. I asked them first to take their pulses and to calculate their heart rates, explaining that rapid heart rate is one response to stress, and that perhaps they would be able to see a measurable benefit from our next activity.

Modified Body Scan Exercise

This exercise is based on one used in the program of the Stress Reduction Clinic at the University of Massachusetts Medical Center, explained in detail in Chapter 5 of Jon Kabat-Zinn's book, *Full Catastrophe Living–Using the Wisdom of Your Body and Mind to Face Stress, Pain, and Illness* (Kabat-Zinn, 1990, p. 76). Kabat-Zinn describes the body-scan as a "very powerful technique we use to reestablish contact with the body. . . Because of the thorough and minute focus on the body in body scanning, it is an effective technique for developing both concentration and flexibility of attention at the same time." The described technique requires the practitioner to lie on a mat on the floor on one's back, with eyes closed. This seemed too demanding given the high level of anxiety, and so I modified the body scan to allow students to remain seated, and to keep the lights on and their eyes open if they wished. (These modifications were validated a week later by an E-mail communiqué from Bobbie Clennell, an Iyenger Yoga teacher in New York, who obtained from Rajvi Mehta a special sequence of yoga asanas that had been used by yoga teachers responding to the earthquake in India in 2000). The specific advice given was: "The emotional strength in these students needs to be built up. No standing poses or backbends. Poses should be done with the eyes open, the gaze soft, focusing inward. Ask the students to imagine that their eyes are located at the temples and ask them to 'open' these eyes. Do not insist on a perfect pose in the current situation" (Mehta, 2002, p. 16).

The body scan is a guided attention exercise. The listeners are told to attend first to their position and to find a comfortable one. Attention is then directed to the breath, and to the tidal motion of the breath that will move on its own without our conscious control or direction. The scan itself then travels from the toes of the left foot slowly up the foot and leg "feeling the sensations as we go and directing the breath to and from the different regions" (Kabat-Zinn, 1990, p. 77). Scanning then proceeds from the right toes up to the pelvis, then through the torso, the back and arms and chest and shoulders, next to the fingers of both hands and up the arms to the shoulders again. Next, the scan moves to the face and the back and top of the head, ending with an image of "breathing through an imaginary 'hole' in the very top of the head, as if we were a whale with a blowhole" (Kabat-Zinn, 1990, p. 77). In the end, the breath is experienced throughout the body, with many practitioners feeling that their bodies have "dropped away or become transparent" (Kabat-Zinn, 1990, p. 77).

Technical Points

Technique is critical to the success of guided relaxation. Points to consider include pacing, use of silence, voice quality, and images suggested. Pacing is generally slow, with pauses to allow practitioners to process, integrate, explore, and experience what their guide is suggesting. Voice quality should be confident and calm, measured and soft while still audible to all present. Selection of images must consider whether all practitioners would be familiar with the given image (an issue in multicultural New York), with an eye to avoiding images that may suggest danger or anything alarming to any of those present (for example, some people find the ocean frightening).

I modified the body scan to suit the situation, and because I did not have the text for the exercise with me, I ad-libbed based on experience teaching yoga-based relaxation. The following are some examples of the suggestions I recall using during the exercise on September 12. The examples are given in the order they would have occurred, but represent only a small sample of the entire exercise, which took about 30 minutes.

- "Find a comfortable and open position, with arms and legs relaxed and uncrossed. . . It may help to let your hands rest in your lap, with palms up. . ."
- "Some people find it works better to close their eyes. But you can keep them open if you feel like it. . . Let your eyes be soft and feel them sink back. Let your eyelids be heavy."
- "Observe your skin, and let your skin soften. . . Let it rest on your body. . . Let the skin be loose and soft."
- "Feel your breath. . . feel how your breath moves in and out of your body. . . focus on the movement of your ribs. Notice that your breath moves on its own. . . no need to supervise it. . . it is there to sustain you."
- After moving up the leg, "bring the breath now to your left knee, and invite the breath to explore your knee, allowing it to move deep into the knee. . . focus on the top and bottom of the knee. . . the inside and outside of the knee. . . consider your knee and only your knee, using the breath. . . "

Results of the Body Scan Exercise

During the body scan exercise, the group remained so still that the lights went off automatically when the sensors failed to detect any movement in the room. As we processed the exercise afterwards, students remarked on feeling much more relaxed than they had prior to the exercise. One student whose heart rate had been 108 beats per minute at the start of the exercise had a rate of 72 beats per minute at the end. Another student described "really feeling my body, feeling different parts getting warm" when the breath was directed to them. Most significant to me, later in the semester, students spontaneously remarked that they had continued to use the exercise on their own to reduce stress, and that it was helpful.

Following the body scan, we did a third activity, finger-painting.

Finger-Painting

Finger-painting is taught in Introduction to Occupational Therapy, which students had completed the previous semester. I explained that we would use finger-painting to explore art as an expressive medium in times of stress. Each student had a half sheet of finger-paint paper and three primary colors of finger-paint (red, blue, yellow). We stood around two tall rectangular workbenches, with room for all to work while facing inwards toward the rest of the group. The directions given were minimal, and deliberately vague and open-ended. "You can paint something specific, or you can explore the paint with your fingers and make shapes. Whatever you do will be all right."

Students worked silently for about 15 minutes. When everyone was finished and cleaned up, I asked the students to walk around and look at each other's work. I then asked if anyone would like to talk about his or her painting. One student had painted a house surrounded by lush flowers and vegetation; she said this was her hope for the future for herself, her husband and child. Another student painted a butterfly and said that this represented hope that something good could come. Some paintings had religious elements. Several others were swirled mixed colors with no particular pattern; one student volunteered that this expressed confusion and fear.

We spent a few minutes connecting this finger-painting event to students' experience in the Introduction to Occupational Therapy course. Several remarked that today's activity had much more meaning and that they could now understand the therapeutic value of the medium. This gave me the opportunity to introduce the theoretical perspective of object relations and connect this experience to the current course work. I am referring here to the psychodynamic model of occupational therapy which uses activities to explore and understand the psychological needs of the client with regard to image of self, concept of others, ego organization, unconscious conflicts and communication (Fidler & Fidler, 1963; Stein & Cutler, 2002). Additional information on the use of art activities to access unconscious material can be found in the text, *Activities: Reality and Symbol* (Fidler & Velde, 1999).

Final Discussion

We gathered in a circle for a final discussion. Some of the topics were:

- Which of the activities was most helpful to you?
- Which one did you like the most? The least?
- Do you think you would try any of these again? Or use them with clients or consumers?
- How are you feeling now? Is there anything further you would like to share? And what are your plans for the next two days?

LIFE AT THE COLLEGE–CONTINUED

Writing retrospectively it is difficult to reconstruct the exact sequence of events, but sometime in early- or mid-October anthrax-tainted mail was reported first in Florida, then in Washington, and in New York. An already tense New York City was further stressed by this new threat. Students almost daily came to me with tears in their eyes to discuss one problem or another. Some of these were normal problems of living experienced as much more critical in the context of the New York and Washington attacks, the Pennsylvania crash, the anthrax-tainted mail, and the air war in Afghanistan (which began on October 7).

The student who had seen the people jumping from the towers was continually in distress, and trying to put up a brave front. Another student, from Uzbekistan, was worried about her mother who lives only a few miles from the Afghan border. She told me that she would never tell her mother about the problems here, because she did not want to upset her and get her worrying. By October 22, it seemed time to try another stress-management exercise in class. This time I adapted one from the Wellness Reproductions Exercises in the *Life Management Skills Workbooks* (Korb-Khalsa & Leutenberg, 1996), "Letter to a Feeling." The original exercise is entitled "Right to Heal: Letter of a Trauma Survivor" (Korb-Khalsa & Leutenberg, 1996, p. 20).

I introduced the activity by asking students to name the negative and stressful feelings they were experiencing. Some identified were fear, anger, sadness, and anxiety. The directions given were to write a letter to the feeling, beginning with "Dear (feeling)." The letter was to include "what the feeling is doing to you, and how it is affecting your life," and to end with "something that you want to know, or a request you want to make." About ten minutes was given to write this letter, with a reminder to the students to sign their names.

Students then were then asked to take a second piece of paper, and write a letter from the feeling to themselves. They were to take the feeling's point of view and honestly try to answer the questions or statements of the first letter. Again, this portion took about ten minutes, but most students finished in five.

I assured students that they did not have to read their letters aloud, but that we would like to listen if anyone cared to do so. All but a few students read. One example: a student from Guyana had been separated from her young daughter (who remained in Guyana with the student's mother) while the student was attending school in New York. She wrote "Dear Sadness, I have never known you before in my life," and went on to express her misery over the separation. In the letter from Sadness to herself, Sadness wrote, "I am sorry I took over your life. You were once someone who was always smiling, now most times you are not" (quoted with permission of Shelly Gomes, OTA student).

Once all those who wished to read had a chance to do so (I also read from my letter "Dear Fear"), I asked students to take a third sheet of paper and write their response to this exercise (five minutes) and we then discussed these responses.

Results of "Letter to a Feeling" Exercise

The most common response was a feeling of surprise that the exercise was so transforming in reducing painful feelings and allowing them to be expressed. Some students had cried during the exercise, both while writing and while reading aloud. Another response made by one student, but echoed by the nods of others was something to the effect that "I did not realize that these feelings were a part of me. I kept pushing them away. Now I understand them better and I see that I can deal with them."

Here is an example from one student: "I think this exercise helped me to look at life more realistically and to face the obstacles that are always in the path of life. This exercise is good too because it helped me to cry which I am always trying not to do. Crying can be a therapy because it helps to ease stress" (quoted with permission of Shelly Gomes, OTA student).

Other Aspects of Life at the College

In late September, faculty with counseling backgrounds or experience was asked to volunteer to lead workshops for students to help them deal with the terrorist attacks and the general security threats. I was one of perhaps six or seven faculty and counselors who participated. Of the four workshops I scheduled during October and November, I had a single student participant at only the first workshop. This was the common experience of all the volunteer faculty group leaders. Our general analysis (after the fact) was that students were not likely to come to see a stranger and to participate in a public forum (however small and intimate) but would instead seek someone they already knew, a counselor or a faculty member, to see privately.

CONCLUSIONS

My work with those affected by the World Trade Center attacks was really quite modest in comparison to therapists who have been more on the front lines of mental health care. A community college such as LaGuardia is an occupational wellness zone–a place where thousands of different kinds of people have serious work to do together, on a daily basis, on a regular schedule. To the faculty, this is normal, ordinary work, the work of education. For many of the students, it is extraordinary work, as many of them are the first in their families to earn any kind of college degree. Thus, as a community, the college followed New York City Mayor Guiliani's exhortations during the fall to "get back to normal" and resume normal activities as much as possible.

On a personal level, bearing witness to the attacks in New York City has been intense work. I have listened to countless personal reports from friends and acquaintances who were eyewitnesses, who barely escaped with their lives, who worked "Ground Zero" as firefighters and emergency workers, and whose children were evacuated on September 11th during extreme chaos from the elementary and high schools near the Twin Towers. I have faced my own fears and those of my child. I have listened. I have tried to hear.

On a professional level, I suspect there is much work ahead of us, particularly in communities directly affected by the attacks. Reports of increased substance use and abuse in New York City following the attacks, predictions of further mental health problems for those affected, unknown public health risks from the ash and toxins inhaled by everyone downwind of the site all testify to the continuing risks for physical and mental health. On the other hand, the courage and determination of the "new" normal suggest that we are designing strategies to cope, and to endure.

REFERENCES

Fidler, G. S. & Fidler, J. W. (1963). *Occupational therapy: A communication process in psychiatry.* New York: Macmillan.

Fidler, G. S. & Velde, B. P. (1999). *Activities: Reality and symbol.* Thorofare, NJ: SLACK.

Kabat-Zinn, J. (1990). *Full catastrophe living–Using the wisdom of your body and mind to face stress, pain, and illness.* New York: Dell Books, pp. 76-77.

Korb-Khalsa, K. & Leutenberg, E. (1996). *Life management skills IV: Reproducible activity handouts created for facilitators.* Plainview, NY: Wellness Reproductions, p. 20.

Mehta, R. (2002). A special sequence of poses. *Yoga Samachar, 6,* 16.

Stein, F. & Cutler, S. K. (2002). *Psychosocial occupational therapy: A holistic approach.* Albany, NY: Delmar Publishing.

Rebuilding Lives Through
the Employment Placement Program
of 9/11

Pat Precin, MS, OTR/L
Chelle Marie, MSW

ECONOMIC IMPACT OF 9/11 ON NEW YORK CITY

The September 11 terrorist attacks on the World Trade Center brought about a vast and completely unprecedented level of impact on the United States. Approximately 3,000 lives were lost as a direct result of the attack, and the number of individuals affected emotionally and financially was enormous and incalculable. In addition to those who lost their lives or were injured, tens of thousands of individuals witnessed the events and aftermath directly, provided rescue relief, lost friends and/or family, lost their homes and/or lost their livelihoods.

New York City lost 131,300 jobs in 2001, one of the largest declines on record. Two-thirds (84,000) of these losses occurred between September 12 and December (Fiscal Policy Institute, March, 2002). The estimates for the total number of jobs lost as a result of September 11 range between 110,000-150,000 (United Way of New York City, 2002). The impact of these attacks extended far beyond Lower Manhattan, and caused economic hardship to those whose jobs depended on travel, tourism, hospitality, and transportation. Low-wage workers were par-

[Haworth co-indexing entry note]: "Rebuilding Lives Through the Employment Placement Program of 9/11." Precin, Pat, and Chelle Marie. Co-published simultaneously in *Occupational Therapy in Mental Health* (The Haworth Press, Inc.) Vol. 21, No. 3/4, 2006, pp. 107-119; and: *Healing 9/11: Creative Programming by Occupational Therapists* (ed: Pat Precin) The Haworth Press, Inc., 2006, pp. 107-119. Single or multiple copies of this article are available for a fee from The Haworth Document Delivery Service [1-800-HAWORTH, 9:00 a.m. - 5:00 p.m. (EST). E-mail address: docdelivery@haworthpress.com].

ticularly affected. According to data collected by the Fiscal Policy Institute (September 2001 and November 2001), every industry except construction experienced job loss. The employment losses in the higher paying industries of securities, insurance, and computer technology were largely a result of jobs relocating out of New York City (thus constituting a job loss to the City, but not to the individual) whereas job losses in other industries largely consisted of layoffs and major reductions in work hours (thus affecting the individual worker). The findings of the Fiscal Policy Institute (March, 2002 and September, 2001) closely mirrored those of the Ground Zero Report (United Way of New York City, 2002) which identified the following major industries as most affected by September 11: retail and wholesale trade which lost 15,200 jobs, food service (12,500), air transport (10,800), the hotel industry (3,500), building services (3,200), and temporary services (2,200). Sixty percent of affected workers had an average wage of $11.00 per hour or $22,000 per year (Eisenberg et al., 2001). As late as June 2002, 40 percent of those who had worked in or around Ground Zero (which does not include airline personnel) were still unemployed (9/11 United Services Group, 2002).

This event also had an impact on the economy of the United States. The cost to the American economy is calculated to be at least ten times greater than the physical damage caused by the attack (Eisenberg et al., 2001). One point four trillion dollars in investor wealth was lost as the Dow Jones industrial average lost 14,000 points (a 14 percent drop) in the weeks following September 11 (Eisenberg et al., 2001).

Unfortunately, individuals who lost their jobs as a result of 9/11, but did not live or work around Ground Zero were ineligible for services or financial assistance from most government and human service providers (9/11 United Services Group, 2002 and United Way of New York City, 2002). An estimated 50,000 workers lost their jobs as a result of 9/11 but were ineligible for assistance (United Way of New York City, 2002). As of February 2002, only 1,800 households had received mortgage and rental assistance (United Way of New York City, 2002). The Federal Emergency Management Agency (FEMA), the American Red Cross, Safe Horizon, and the Salvation Army focused their efforts on individuals who lived or worked south of Canal Street (FEMA later expanded their geographic parameters to cover the entire island of Manhattan) and who could document that they had lost their jobs because of 9/11. As a result, individuals who had lived and worked in the boroughs outside of Manhattan (displaced airline workers in particular) were not able to receive assistance, or were independent contractors such as limousine drivers, or undocumented immigrants.

BROOKLYN BUREAU OF COMMUNITY SERVICE'S COMMUNITY RESPONSE CENTER

The Brooklyn Bureau of Community Service is a not-for-profit organization that has been dedicated to helping under-served residents of Brooklyn, New York maximize their functioning in the community for the last 137 years. With over 30 different programs in the areas of family, psychiatric, and adult rehabilitation services, and over 700 employees from different professional disciplines and support staff, the Bureau is consistently able to provide new services to its community as appropriate.

In response to the disastrous events of 9/11, BBCS rapidly developed and implemented the Community Response Center (CRC) to provide financial assistance, employment placement, and case management services for those who lost their jobs as a direct or residual effect of 9/11. The CRC was funded by the following: The New York Times 9/11 Neediest Fund, McCormick Tribune Foundation Disaster Relief Fund, Robin Hood Relief Fund, The Junior League Disaster Relief Fund, AIG Disaster Relief Fund, Coalition of Voluntary Mental Health Agencies, The September 11th Fund, Rockefeller Brothers Fund, International Paper Company Employee Relief Fund, International Paper Company Foundation, The US Jaycees, The Starr Foundation, Chances for Children, Pittsburgh Pirate Wives Charities, Brooklyn Heights Synagogue, Advent Lutheran Church, Chandhok Charitable Trust, Stroock Spirit of New York Fund, First Church of Christ Scientist, Stuart Four Square Fund, James and Elizabeth Hughes Foundation, and The Society for the Promotion of Japanese Animation.

The CRC initially served all those who were affected by 9/11. The Brooklyn Bureau shifted its focus to provide financial assistance primarily to those who worked north of Canal Street or outside of Manhattan because they were not eligible for services from the Red Cross, Salvation Army, or Safe Horizon. The CRC continues to provide other services including case management, counseling, and employment services to all persons affected by 9/11. This chapter describes the strategies used by the authors (first author, Acting Coordinator, second author, Coordinator) to develop and implement the Employment Placement Program (EPP) of the CRC.

Clientele

At its peak, the EPP was serving 400 people per week. Most had worked in the towers or the immediate area, had witnessed the event, and were evacuated without injury. They were dealing with the initial horror and trauma, grief, terror, shock, and loss of their friends and co-workers. Others who did not go into work that day saw the attack on television and knew their workplace had been destroyed and their friends and coworkers were quite possibly dead. They were horrified and particularly devastated by their inability to help. Many clients faced emotional trauma, financial ruin, and major life disruption all at one time, and did not know what to address first. For many, their last pay-check was all they had and they received no severance pay. Living in such an expensive city, paycheck to paycheck, many had no savings and were unable to pay rent and bills, or otherwise provide for themselves. Many were coming to a charity for the first time in their lives.

As a result, many clients had psychological issues such as fear, anxiety, depression, sleep disorders, substance abuse, Post Traumatic Stress Disorder (PTSD), and traumatic grief, that needed to be addressed before seeking employment.

The literature reports that 70 percent of workers whose employment was affected by 9/11, were members of minority groups, predominately Hispanic and Chinese (9/11 United Service Group, 2002). The EPP also had a high preponderance of immigrant clientele. Immigrants are more prone to experience symptoms of PTSD due to memories of terrorism, war, or violence possibly experienced in their country of origin. Those who are "out of status" or "undocumented" do not have legal status to reside and/or work in the United States. There is a great deal of uncertainty regarding what services are available. Many will not seek or accept services because they fear that the service provider will report them, resulting in deportation. The Immigration Reform Act of 1996 and part of the Welfare Reform Act both indicate that a person's eligibility for his/her citizenship status would be affected if he/she utilized public assistance. As a result, legal immigrants often fear that utilizing other public and nonprofit services including employment placement programs, may hinder their ability to attain full citizenship.

Many clients had children who experienced difficulty in school due to anxiety, physical symptoms, lowered self-esteem, academic difficulties, social problems, aggressive and defiant behaviors, depression, grief or PTSD as a result of 9/11, and consequently needed extra time and resources to help them.

Most clients were former employees of the airline, administrative/office, housekeeping, transportation, food service, media and communication, or computer industries (Table 1).

PHASES OF THE EMPLOYMENT PLACEMENT PROGRAM

The strategy for the EPP can be broken up into two phases. Phase I resembled the private industry employment agency structure that emphasizes placing the largest number of people as quickly as possible. Phase II utilized an employment counseling services model. However, before Phase I could begin, a Pre-Phase was necessary to allow clients to express their emotions and experiences about 9/11 in a group setting.

Pre-Phase

In order to expedite services, the EPP program began in another BBCS employment service program, PRIDE. The EPP was able to utilize PRIDE's staff, computers, and group rooms in the evenings and on weekends (after PRIDE's hours of operation) to establish a job bank and hire their own staff while servicing the hundreds of clients who were being referred.

Initially, EPP clients were emotionally raw and needed to discuss their feelings and experiences with others who had had similar experiences before they could concentrate on job search. Group settings with experienced leaders provided a forum for people to express themselves, empathize, problem solve and share outside resources until they were ready for Phase I. At each meeting, after discussion, clients were assisted to prepare updated resumes. Anyone requiring additional psychosocial services was referred to another program within BBCS.

Later, EPP secured its own space, which was large enough to service the expanding program.

Phase I

Rapidly moving the most employable candidates into jobs decreased caseloads down to a manageable size and enabled staff to concentrate on providing more individualized and comprehensive services to their remaining clients. This was both a necessary and effective method for numerous reasons. The employment team came on board with an existing caseload that was unmanageable any other way. Each placement

TABLE 1. CRC Employment Statistics from 09/11/2001 to 09/11/2002

Employment Type	# of Clients with Previous Employment	# of Clients Employed
Administrative/Office	458	23
Airline	718	49
Beauty/Fashion	34	2
Computer Professions	152	6
Construction	13	5
Customer Service	7	4
Education	23	2
Employment Services	9	0
Engineering	7	1
Financial Services	100	8
Food Service	227	14
Garment Industry	10	0
Health and Human Services	43	17
Hotel	77	7
Hotel (Not Housekeeping)	65	5
Housekeeping (Hotel)	381	31
Housekeeping/Janitorial (Not Hotel)	73	10
Manufacturing and Production	56	3
Media and Communications	153	7
Retail or Other Sales	149	9
Security/Public Safety/Legal Services	79	10
Transportation	300	29
Travel and Tourism	113	0
Unclassified/Other	320	20

specialist had well over 200 cases at a time when a program structure was not fully implemented and there was an absolute dearth of jobs. Many recipients did not need in-depth employment counseling or job readiness training, since at the time of the attack they had been employed. Their top need was job leads, not employment readiness preparation. Those with greater skills and educational levels obtained employment sooner.

The following five elements were key to the strategy of the EPP.

The first element was recruiting staff with the highest possible caliber of private industry experience and connections. All Employment Placement Specialists were private sector recruiters drawn from the business, news media/information technology, hospitality, and financial sectors. A significant amount of time was placed on recruitment. It was critical to hire staff with significant experience, intelligence, and motivation for these positions, as in addition to performing employment placement they would be co-developing and implementing a program. In order to assure that the most up-to-date methods of placement services would be used in the program, emphasis was place on identifying applicants who had worked for high volume placement agencies.

The second key element was the use of an incentive system for placements. Placement Specialists were offered a base salary with an additional amount of money given for each placement they made over a certain number.

Third, heavy use of volunteers, with particular emphasis on those with significant private sector experience. Volunteers providing workshops on resume development and interviewing skills included a business development associate from JP Morgan and several Human Resource associates from major corporations and executive placement services.

The fourth key element was conducting a program strategy with assistance from business management consultants. Private sector executives were more than willing to provide assistance in response to such a catastrophic event. Business executives, including senior executives of management consulting firms and corporations in multiple sectors, were forthcoming with providing assistance free of charge when approached.

The fifth key element: heavy use of technology, particularly for staff recruitment, data management, and acquisition and disbursement of job leads. Information technology experts generously provided their assistance free of charge in response to this disaster. Particular use was made of database developers and management experts. Additionally, computer expertise was a critical skill for all staff involved in the project.

Technology proved to be beneficial on multiple levels. All program staff was recruited using online employment resources in addition to the newspaper. The use of online employment resources provided a screening mechanism, such that only applicants with at least a moderate level of computer expertise utilized this method. The overall caliber of the applicants who responded to the online job postings was significantly higher than those who responded to our newspaper advertisement. In addition, the high volume of resumes received through these sources (monster.com in particular) was both beneficial and time consuming. The primary benefit was that we were able to be highly selective; the disadvantage was that the number of resumes received was enormous (300 within a few hours of posting the position), thus a great deal of time was consumed reviewing resumes. This time was well invested; however, as we were able to hire highly qualified and competent staff.

Once the staff was hired, the employment placement team made extensive use of technology to rapidly develop and implement an effective program. It was fully operational within one month of its inception and, by the end of that first month, the staff had not only met their employment placement goals, they more than doubled them. By September 11, 2002, EPP had provided employment services to 624 individuals.

These outcomes were achieved as a result of effective utilization of technology, the private industry experience staff members brought with them, and the collaboration involved in both developing strategies and procedures and providing direct services.

The ways in which technology was used creatively are as follows:

- *Creation of industry specific E-mail accounts linked to employment web sites:* Over 20 E-mail accounts were created and linked to 100 web sites that automatically forwarded job leads to an E-mail account categorized by industry and by specified criteria for the type of position sought. For example, an E-mail account was created for entry level and senior level secretarial positions and that email address was registered with all of the employment sites that generated secretarial postings. Another E-mail account for security positions was set up and linked that email address to the appropriate web sites, and so forth. These web sites generated job leads on a daily or weekly basis. Placement specialists were given the E-mail user name (the name of the account) and password for these accounts, and were assigned specific accounts that they were required to check daily. Setting up a separate account for each industry (rather than creating one account that generated leads in multiple industries) alleviated the need to sort through the job leads and enabled staff and clients to rapidly access leads in the industries of interest to them. Setting up each account took 30 minutes. Linking these accounts to the job web sites took three people only two days.

- *Dissemination of job leads:* The employment placement specialists obtained job leads which they shared among themselves and distributed to the clients, using a variety of techniques, mainly involving computer technology. The employment placement specialists checked the E-mail accounts assigned to them, and forwarded appropriate leads to the clients on their caseload either by phone or E-mail. This process took a few hours per day, yet was significantly more efficient than printing leads and inserting them into a binder that clients need to come on site to view. It was also more efficient and effective than mailing the job leads. The Employment Placement Specialists showed those clients who did not already have E-mail accounts how to set up free accounts for themselves, which they then accessed through computers on site or via other computers to which they had access.

The EPP set up a shared directory using Groupwise. Folders in different industries were set up and job leads from multiple sources (online, E-mail accounts, networking with employers, and leads obtained through job fairs) were forwarded into these folders. All placement specialists accessed these folders to view job leads.

Separate folders for resumes in different industries were also created on the network's shared drive and all staff instantly accessed the resumes for all clients in a given field of employment, regardless of who was on their caseload. The staff then matched the clients with job leads. Use of the database for client matching had been the program's original intent but proved to be more difficult. Instead, a system of storing resumes was simple to implement and took less than a half-hour to create, and a matter of moments to store them. Because this was set up through E-mail, job leads were forwarded to clients instantly.

This method of job lead acquisition and disbursement was very efficient and saved on paper. The biggest limitation of this approach was that obtaining a job through online leads is quite difficult in a city as large and competitive as New York. Thousands of applicants may compete for one open position. Thus, clients had to respond to a job posting immediately because an employer may become saturated with resumes within a day.

An internal contact is almost always more effective than a response to a blind ad, so Employment Placement Specialists balanced their time between online job sourcing, employer outreach, cold calling (in person and over the phone), networking at job fairs, networking through attendance at conferences, and direct promotion of individual clients through targeted mailings to select employers.

• *Client data management.* A vast amount of data was collected, tracked, processed, and shared for this program on a Microsoft Access database. The database was divided into 11 separate sections: client demographic information, employment history, office visits, services provided, financial disbursements given, referrals made, employer contact information, candidate status with employers (interview given, resume sent, and placement made) follow up and outreach information, computer class registration and course completion, and progress notes. Reports were generated to track demographics, outcomes, trends, staff performance, and services provided for any specified period of time. Although extremely helpful, developing and maintaining such an extensive database required a great deal of skill and knowledge. Programs wishing to develop and maintain a highly comprehensive database must have staff willing and knowledgeable enough to use such a system, adequate technical support and sufficiently powerful computing and networking hardware.

Phase II

The second phase of the program utilized an employment counseling model, shifting the goals for the Employment Placement Specialists from linking the maximum number of people with jobs to providing in depth services to each client on their caseload. Greater emphasis was placed on assessing barriers to employment, candidate needs, vocational interests and aptitudes, and on long-term career planning. This presented a challenge because none of the Specialists had worked with this model before. Changing focus required adaptation. The two-phase model enabled this shift because the Specialists' caseloads were greatly reduced after the first round of candidates obtained employment. Having devoted time to the program, strong relationships existed with the remaining candidates.

Those who remained unemployed for a long period of time needed more intensive services, either because their inability to obtain employment was, to a certain extent, related to barriers that required more in-depth assistance, or because the effect of being unemployed in and of itself began producing obstacles that would need to be addressed with greater depth. Individuals who were already in a risky financial situation were in an increasingly desperate position due to the fact that unemployment insurance provided only half of already low wages and unpaid bills continued to accumulate while they remain unemployed. Many individuals were unable to generate income at their previous level, as they could not find jobs that paid what they had been earning prior to September 11. Of those that had been reemployed by their former employer, approximately 85 percent worked a reduced schedule. The individuals who obtained employment with a new employer usually worked full time, though many received a lower salary than prior to the event. The primary example is housekeepers with high school educations or less and limited English skills, who previously made more than $17 an hour in the hotel industry and now receive $10 an hour or less cleaning private homes.

The two-phase model provided two major benefits to the CRC program. A large number of people were provided assistance with a very short turn-around time. At its peak volume in Phase I, financial assistance was provided within one-to-three days, with the majority of assistance provided on the day the client sought services. Also, a large number of people were provided employment assistance, and obtained employment (see Table I for a list of jobs that people have obtained through the EPP), in a relatively short period of time.

OBSTACLES TO IMPLEMENTATION

There were many difficulties in implementing the EPP. The 9/11 tragedy presented unique challenges for the staff. Most critical was its magnitude; the staff was swamped with hundreds of needy individuals all at one time, needing services that they were not initially prepared to deliver. Many staff members were traumatized by the event and were not trained in trauma counseling. The situation, rather than the client, presented the "problem." A lot of social service programs exist to help individuals change in order to function more effectively in their environment. For employment programs, this usually entails job readiness assistance and for mental health services, it often means helping people with preexisting, long-term psychiatric disorders to improve their functioning. For this program, the job seekers were not "the problem," the lack of jobs was; a preexisting "psychiatric disorder" was not the problem, an unexpected terrorist attack was.

The CRC's goal had been to meet the urgent needs of the participants for placement and financial assistance, but this did not meet the long-term needs of the participants who might require retraining and assistance to transition into growth industries in which they could earn a more viable income, advance, and receive full benefits.

CONCLUSION

The McKinsey report (9/11 United Services Group, 2002) estimates that the primary needs of those affected by 9/11 are: financial assistance, mental health, job training and placement, childcare, eldercare, language training, and children's education. They further estimate that 90 percent of the need for assistance is concentrated among affected workers (workers that lost their jobs as a result of 9/11). A large percentage of funding for 9/11 has been targeted for economic revitalization and assistance to family members of those who died in the event, but the largest gap of unmet financial need is among the surviving affected workers (9/11 United Service Group, 2002). These workers are the people to whom BBCS's EPP is dedicated and will continue to be dedicated to servicing through gainful employment.

REFERENCES

9/11 United Services Group (2002, June). *A study of the ongoing needs of people affected by the World Trade Center disaster: Key findings and recommendations.* New York, NY: Study conducted by McKinsey & Co. Retrieved on June 15, 2002, from http://www.9-11usg.org/index3.asp?page=REPSTUDIDX#critical.

Eisenberg, D., Donnelly, S., Thompson, M., Tumulty, K., Weisskopf, M., Baumohl, B. et al. (2001, October). Wartime Recession? *Time Atlantic, 158* (14), 58.

Fiscal Policy Institute. (2001, September) *Economic impact of the September 11 World Trade Center attack: Preliminary report.* (Prepared for the New York City Central Labor Council and the Consortium for Worker Education). New York, NY. Retrieved June 15, 2002 from http://www.fiscalpolicy.org/sep28WTCreport.pdf.

Fiscal Policy Institute. (2001, November). *World Trade Center job impacts take a heavy toll on low wage workers: Occupational and wage implications of job losses related to the September 11 World Trade Center attack.* (Prepared for the New York City Central Labor Council and the Consortium for Worker Education). New York, NY. Retrieved June 15, 2002 from http://www.fiscalpolicy.org/Nov5WTCreport.PDF.

Fiscal Policy Institute. (2002, March). *The employment impact of the September 11 World Trade Center attacks: Updated estimates based on the benchmarked employment data.* New York, NY. Retrieved on June 15, 2002, from http://www. fiscalpolicy.org/Employment%20Impact%20of%20September%2011_Update.pdf.

United Way of New York City. (2002, March). *Beyond Ground Zero: Challenges and implications for human services in New York City post September 11.* New York, NY: Report prepared by Appleseed, Inc. Retrieved June 15, 2002 from http://www. uwnyc.org/640/.

RESOURCES

Assessment tool: Horowitz, M., Wilner, N.J. & Alvarez, W. (1979) Impact of events scale: A measure of subjective stress. *Psychosomatic Medicine,* 41, 209-218.

Information scientist: Fred Lerner, D.L.S. National Center for Post-Traumatic Stress Disorder, VA Medical Center (116D), White River Junction, Vermont 05009. Phone (802) 296-5132. Fax (802) 296-5135. Internet: fred.lerner@dartmouth.edu.

The International Society for Traumatic Stress Studies: http://www.istss.org.

The National Center for PTSD: Comprehensive information about different assessment instruments to use with those affected by trauma. (802) 296-6300 http://www. ncptsd.org.

The PTSD Research Quarterly. The PILOTS database is an electronic index to the worldwide literature on post-traumatic stress disorder (PTSD) and other mental-health consequences of exposure to traumatic events. It is produced by the National Center for PTSD, and is available to the public on computer systems maintained by Dartmouth College. There is no charge for using the database, and no account or password is required. As of 28 July 2002, there were 21,966 references (almost all including abstracts) in the database. Direct quote from the National Center for PTSD.

Occupational Therapist, Biomedical Science Corps Officer and Former Firefighter

Frank R. Pascarelli, OTR/L, NMS, CPI

INTRODUCTION

I remember the day as if it were yesterday. It was 0900 Eastern Time; I was pulling out of my driveway on my way to a meeting at Children's Healthcare of Atlanta, Georgia. I just turned on the radio news and heard with disbelief that a plane had crashed into the World Trade Center in New York City. I quickly got onto my cell phone and called the Command Post at Dobbins Air Reserve Base. I reached a former colleague, Staff Sergeant Wendy Giles, and headed out to the base. Wendy and I sat in the command post watching the situation unfold when a second plane hit the other tower. Almost immediately, the Command Post Console lit up like a Christmas tree. I received a call from BG Busbee, the commander of 22nd Air Force, instructing us to go to Threatcon Delta. It was at that moment I knew we were at war. Not since the Japanese Bombing of Pearl Harbor has a foreign entity inflicted a direct attack on American soil. Within hours, the base, which has a relatively high level of security, was essentially closed to all except for essential personnel. Cobb County Police and Sheriff Department along with the

[Haworth co-indexing entry note]: "Occupational Therapist, Biomedical Science Corps Officer and Former Firefighter." Pascarelli, Frank R. Co-published simultaneously in *Occupational Therapy in Mental Health* (The Haworth Press, Inc.) Vol. 21, No. 3/4, 2006, pp. 121-128; and: *Healing 9/11: Creative Programming by Occupational Therapists* (ed: Pat Precin) The Haworth Press, Inc., 2006, pp. 121-128. Single or multiple copies of this article are available for a fee from The Haworth Document Delivery Service [1-800-HAWORTH, 9:00 a.m. - 5:00 p.m. (EST). E-mail address: docdelivery@haworthpress.com].

Marietta Police Department assisted in external security until Air Force Security Forces could be mustered.

I remember when leaving the base and driving south on I-75 on my way to Children's Healthcare of Atlanta, there was an eerie sense of quiet above the skies, as a result of the Federal Aviation Administration grounding all commercial and personal aircraft. I arrived to find the meeting postponed as staff desperately sought to gain information on the event. Like all freedom loving people, the staff was experiencing unsettling feelings and emotions. Staff members were crying and clinging to one another for support.

Several hours later, the Children's Healthcare of Atlanta Team answered the call from the Red Cross to donate blood. Their response served two important purposes. It ensured an adequate blood supply for the victims of the attacks, and it gave the rest of America an opportunity to help the victims. One of the worst feelings people experience in a crisis situation is that of helplessness. Empowerment helps people cope with disaster.

CALLED TO DUTY

As a Biomedical Science Corps Officer in the Air Force Reserves, I knew I would be called in to assist. I was in daily contact with Lt. Col. Dan Stoutt, Flight Commander Surgical Operations Squadron 96th Medical Group at Eglin Air Force Base and in frequent contact with the Director of Health Professions Office of The Surgeon General in Denver. Lt. Col. Stoutt sent me to New York to conduct a needs assessment and to provide crisis intervention. No one on the plane spoke on my way to New York, especially as we flew over Manhattan. When I landed, I knew things had changed; the entire airport had significant numbers of armed federal officers, and they checked everything.

As I crossed over the George Washington Bridge from New Jersey, and drove down to New York City, it too had changed. There were roadblocks and security checkpoints set up along the West Side Drive. Even the checkpoints I experienced in West Germany following the United States bombing on Libya in 1986 did not compare to this. For the first time in 43 years, I did not feel like a New Yorker. The place where I grew up had changed forever. The terrorists attacked the World Trade Center, but the amount of collateral damage was indescribable.

My first assignment was to work at the Family Support Center (FSC) in the Mental Health Section. The center was set up for families, friends and anyone else that needed assistance for most anything concerning the attack on New York. There were representatives from every federal, state, and local agency that could provide assistance.

I treated mostly children whose school had been located in the shadows of the World Trade Center. I used drawings with the children and their family members as a diagnostic tool as drawing is an unstructured projective method of assessment that taps into its creator's conscious and unconscious mental functioning. The drawings provided by the children at the FSC helped to understand their stressors, emotional, social, and cognitive functioning. The process of making art, the product produced and the verbal associations to it may be used to help the individual's inner experience as they are reflected in the process, form and content of the work. I also used drawing as a method of helping the children re-experience their conflicts and resolve them.

The children who attended school near Ground Zero expressed their fears and concerns in their drawings by showing their school engulfed in flames. What was once a green oasis among the skyscrapers of Manhattan was now a battlefield of debris. These children experienced the devastating effects of terrorism firsthand. Their main fear was that this would happen again, and that their mother and/or father would not come home from work.

All other children I treated (those who did not live or go to school within close proximity of the World Trade Center) still drew pictures of their school with a plane crashing into it and the building on fire. After completing their drawings, most children were able to verbalize their fears that this would happen to them in their school. Parents also expressed concerns about their ability to provide a sense of security for their children.

Following this traumatic event, many of the children that I worked with displayed at least one if not several of the following responses:

- They feared separations from their parent(s) or caregivers.
- Their behaviors regressed to younger behaviors such as wetting the bed, sucking their thumbs, sleep disturbances, and fear of the dark.
- They cried.
- They withdrew.
- They stopped participating in their normal routine activities.
- They refused to go to school.
- They exhibited difficulty concentrating.
- They complained of stomachaches and headaches.

- They had feelings of guilt.
- They asked the same question over and over again.
- They feared for their own safety.
- They feared their own death.
- They demonstrated a lack of trust.

In order to help the children through their trauma, the following things were done:

- We limited the children's exposure to media.
- We encouraged the children to tell stories or to use other media to express themselves such as puppets.
- We were honest in answering their questions.
- We encouraged the children to discuss their feelings, told them that these feelings are normal and that they are not alone in experiencing them.
- We worked with parents to encourage them to hold their children to provide them comfort, assure their children that they are now safe, keep their children's routines as normal as possible, offer a night light, reassure them that it is all right to cry and that the disaster was not their fault, develop a disaster plan for the home and have a police person, firefighter, or military personnel talk to their children's school or faith based group.

NEW YORKERS EXPRESSING THEMSELVES

New York adults as well as children were expressing themselves through art. Memorials, flags, hats, flowers, altars, posters and other forms of art could be found all over Manhattan. These works of self-expression helped to reduce anxiety and confusion. They allowed individuals who had difficulty communicating verbally an opportunity to express their concerns, feelings, and emotions. This tool is often less threatening to the individual than direct verbal expression.

Other people volunteered to make food and provide other comforts for the workers involved in the rescue and recovery operations. There was a group of a dozen or so people one night standing not far from Ground Zero holding signs thanking the workers (Photos 1-2). I remember making a U-Turn and stopped to thank them. They were just ordinary people out showing their support; however, to me they were extraordinary people. These simple acts of kindness energized our re-

PHOTO 1. People Thanking Ground Zero Workers.

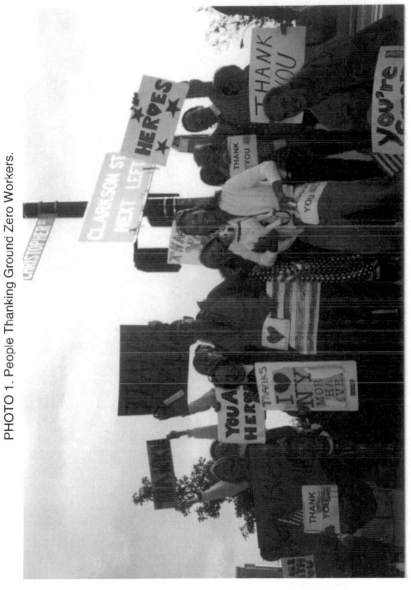

PHOTO 2. A Woman Thanking Ground Zero Workers

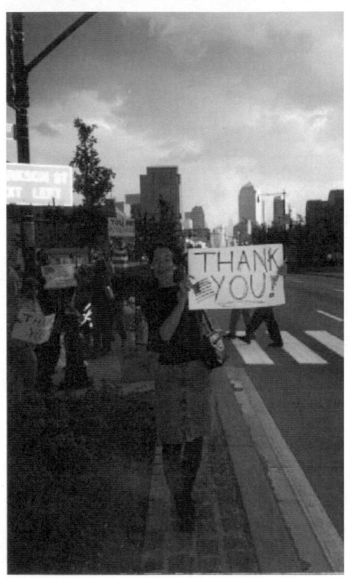

Photo by Frank Pascarelli. Used by permission.

solve in an environment of great despair. These folks were lifting the sprits of those in need back home.

Although New York is some 900 miles away from Atlanta, the inner psyche of Atlanta was affected. Many reservists were activated to fight the war on terror overseas, while others were activated to provide home-land security. Many of the people I have worked with in Atlanta have been experiencing sleep disturbances from anxiety. They were anxious about the safety of their families, their futures, and the possibility that there may be an attack on Atlanta. I remember talking to a chemist that had some realistic fears of what would happen if the terrorists somehow got into the Centers for Disease Control and Prevention and exposed what is in the Level III Lab. A physics professor was concerned about possible attacks on our poorly defended nuclear reactors in Georgia and the rest of the country. These were but just a few of the daily challenges we were facing across the country.

AT EGLIN AIR FORCE BASE

Since the attacks of 9/11, the military has shifted into high gear. One of the things I have been asked to do is provide assessment briefings to mental health professionals on what I saw in New York, and what we could expect from the 18- and 19-year-old soldiers returning from over-seas. Down the road from the Eglin Air Force Base is Hurlber Field, home to the Special Operations Command. (This is from where some of the highest trained war fighters are deployed from.) The mental health staff that serve this community wants to be in a position to address the community's special needs. One psychologist expressed his concern, stating, "We have very good training for mental heath issues in hospi-tals or clinics, but have little or no experience in managing anything like what happened in New York or what these 18- and 19-year-olds experi-enced."

Prior to the events of 9/11, the biggest challenge for many of these single young soldiers was first being the best soldier for their country, then getting a date for Friday night. Now, they were clearing out caves involving direct line of fire in some faraway land called Afghanistan. The numbers are not in yet, but if history repeats itself, there will be an increase in depression and alcohol use as the young combatants return from their overseas missions.

POST 9/11 RECOVERY

As an Occupational Therapist, Air Force Officer and former fire-fighter, I believe there are several things that can help people recover from the events of 9/11. While the site was active, on-site intervention was critical. Now that the site is closed, there continues to be a need for intervention not just to those in New York but also to anyone who feels they need the support. Part of this recognition of support rests with primary care providers. I have been instructing providers to identify clients who need extra support through accurately observing and listening with a third ear for possible unreported signs and symptoms, asking in-depth questions, then making appropriate referrals. Before Occupational Therapists can adequately respond to a mass casualty situation, they need to be both physically and emotionally fit and well versed on how a disaster affects all aspects of the human condition.

Reach Out and Have Some Fun: Combating Isolation in the Aftermath of Terror: A Program for Psychiatric Patients

Cheryl King, MS, OTR

The scene at the psychiatric outpatient program of St. Luke's/Roosevelt Hospital on September 11 was pretty much like any of the other places in New York where people were lucky enough to be out of the direct line of fire. Information trickled in from radios, telephones, and horrified patients and staff members who had seen the towers fall, or had been stuck downtown. Staff and patients desperately tried to locate loved ones and find out more information. Agitated therapists tried to calm patients. As the day wore on, there were tears of relief as friends and relatives were contacted and panic, as the vast number of missing became clear. It was a day when some of the boundaries between patient and therapist blurred and we were all citizens of a stricken New York.

Additionally, during the first days when it was still unknown how many (or few) wounded there would be, our hospital, like other hospitals in the city was on disaster alert. Some of the psychiatry staff was diverted to around the clock emergency room duty to counsel the injured and family members seeking their loved ones. Due to transportation disruptions patients and staff members alike were either unable to get to

[Haworth co-indexing entry note]: "Reach Out and Have Some Fun: Combating Isolation in the Aftermath of Terror: A Program for Psychiatric Patients." King, Cheryl. Co-published simultaneously in *Occupational Therapy in Mental Health* (The Haworth Press, Inc.) Vol. 21, No. 3/4, 2006, pp. 129-143; and: *Healing 9/11: Creative Programming by Occupational Therapists* (ed: Pat Precin) The Haworth Press, Inc., 2006, pp. 129-143. Single or multiple copies of this article are available for a fee from The Haworth Document Delivery Service [1-800- HAWORTH, 9:00 a.m. - 5:00 p.m. (EST). E-mail address: docdelivery@haworthpress.com].

doi:10.1300/J004v21n03_09

work or treatment, or unable to get back home. Many individuals lived in neighborhoods where the sight and the smell of smoke were pervasive. While some patients called or came in for extra support, many more stayed home, too fearful to venture outside.

Over the weeks and months that followed, it became clear that the experiences of September 11 would leave their mark on all New Yorkers. Initial research clearly suggested that many individuals were experiencing depression, anxiety, acute stress reactions, increased substance abuse, and post traumatic stress disorder. Many of our 2,000+ psychiatric outpatients were bound to experience some of these population effects. Specific risk factors for clinical symptomatology began to emerge. We wondered to what extent these were present in our patient population. What would be the additional burden of a major terrorist attack on individuals already suffering from a major mental illness?

This paper will review the research efforts from September 11 and prior terror incidents to identify global reactions and risk factors for increased distress. The demographics of our patient population will be analyzed in light of these general risk factors. Factors that could be sources of additional distress in our seriously mentally ill adult outpatient population will then be discussed. The development and funding of a theoretically based support program open to all of our patients will be described. Finally, the program plans and outcome parameters will be shared.

One source for predicting the types of long term reactions that could be expected to occur after 9/11 was research done in response to the Oklahoma City bombing in 1995. One early finding was that 61.5% of the adults in Oklahoma City reported experiencing at least one direct result of the bombing. When compared to a control group, Oklahomans reported about double the amount of alcohol abuse, double the amount of psychological distress, double the amount of intrusive thoughts related to the bombing, and double the number of Post Traumatic Stress Disorder (PTSD) components. This level of symptomatology persisted for over a year (Smith, Christiansen, Vincent, & Hann, 1999). Predictors of later development of PTSD symptoms included being injured, feeling nervous or afraid at the time of the bombing, reporting that counseling was useful (Tucker, Pfefferbaum, Nixon, & Dickson, 2000), and the development of traumatic grief (Pfefferbaum et al., 2001).

In an unrelated study, negative events occurring before and after two man-made traumatic events (a fire and motor vehicle accidents) were studied as predictors of the development and severity of post traumatic stress disorder (Maes, Mylle, Delmeire, & Janca, 2001). The authors found that there were no significant relationships between stressful life events the year prior to the traumatic events and the development of PTSD. However, the number and severity of stressful events following the traumatic events were highly correlated to the risk of developing PTSD and higher severity of the avoidance-depression dimension of PTSD.

From this literature, we could assume that the two years following the attack would be a critical time for our patients, that they might become increasingly avoidant and increase their substance abuse. The finding that stressful events following a traumatic event were highly correlated to the risk of developing PTSD was particularly relevant in light of the anthrax attacks, repeated public alerts, and an unrelated plane crash that traumatized New Yorkers after the initial attacks.

Rapidly, the initial research reports gauging the reaction to September 11th began appearing. A national survey carried out on September 14th to 16th found that 44% of adults reported one or more substantial symptoms of stress and 90% had one or more symptoms to at least some degree. Their coping strategies included talking with others (90%), turning to religion (90%), and participating in group activities (60%) (Schuster et al., 2001). A study done by members of the Center for Urban Epidemiological Studies of the New York Academy of Medicine (Galea et al., 2002), identified predictors of PTSD and Major Depression five to eight weeks after the attack using a multivariate model. Predictors of PTSD included Hispanic ethnicity, two or more prior stressors, a panic attack during or shortly after the events, residence south of Canal Street, and loss of possessions due to the event. Predictors of Major Depression included Hispanic ethnicity, two or more prior stressors, a panic attack, a low level of social support, the death of a friend or relative during the attacks, and loss of a job.

While many of our patients already suffered from major depression and post traumatic stress, we wanted to ascertain the numbers of patients meeting the risk profiles, as they could be at risk for exacerbation of their illness. Utilizing our Electronic Database, we examined a sample of 274 patients assessed in our Outpatient Access Center from July 1 through September 11 as an estimate of the demographic makeup of our current outpatient census. We were able to determine percentages for race, level of social support, and neighborhood. While we could not determine all past stressors, we did have data for the major traumatic stressors of physical and sexual abuse (see Table 1).

We then reviewed the entries for significant life events on treatment plans for 723 patients completed between September 15, 2001 and Jan-

TABLE 1. Data on 274 Access Center Assessments for Admission to the St. Luke's/Roosevelt Outpatient Psychiatry Programs July 1, 2001-September 11, 2001.

Risk Factor	Percentage
Hispanic ethnicity	35
Low level of social support	48
History of physical abuse	34
History of sexual abuse	27
Residency south of Canal Street	< 1

uary 15, 2002. We found that therapists noted the World Trade Center collapse or the anthrax scare as a stressful event for 35% of the patients. Symptom escalation due to the traumatic events was noted for 6% of the patients. The most prevalent symptom was increase in anxiety followed by increase in isolation. We assume that this measure significantly under reports the degree of stress and symptomatology actually present in our patient population as the field is a standard treatment plan reporting field and no questions or prompts directly addressed the issues of 9/11. Also, given the inarticulate and withdrawn nature of many of our patients and the potential of delayed reactions in response to trauma, the time frame could be too narrow to identify many reactions.

From this data it appeared that the greatest population risk factors for increased distress among our patients included the high percentage of Hispanic patients, the high number of patients with impaired support networks, and the severe degree of trauma in many patients' backgrounds. They also shared with the general population an increased vulnerability to future stressors and a risk for increased smoking and substance abuse.

We were unable to find data sources that detailed risk factors for exacerbation of illness in already mentally ill individuals, although Shuster et al. (2001) in their national study of response to the September 11th attack found that individuals who reported a prior emotional or mental health problem were more likely (p = .05) to report a substantial stress reaction.

The vast majority of our patients already suffered from major mental disorders complicated by social problems, and poor functioning. One of our major models of understanding serious mental illness, the stress diathesis model, seemed to offer a theoretical structure for hypothesizing the scope of the impact the tragedy could have. In general, this model postulates that a genetic, neurocognitive deficit creates a predisposing vulnerability in the form of over-sensitivity to stress. Environmental stress can then precipitate illness. Social support, coping, and competence are intervening variables that can mediate the emergence of illness. In the 1980s, researchers were already studying the impact of life events on the chronically mentally ill. Baker, Burns, Libby, and Intagliata (1985) suggested that life events causing changes over which patients felt no sense of control tended to have stressful consequences, which without preventive intervention could become serious crises. Gordon et al. (1985) developed an algorithm predicting admission to and length of stay on an inpatient unit using data derived from Axis 4 (level of stressors) and Axis 5 (level of functioning) of the Diagnostic and Statistical Manual, Third Edition (American Psychiatric Association, 1980). They computed a strain ratio that is the quotient of the stress score divided by the functional level score. Their results showed that the lower the functional level, the less stress it required to precipitate or prolong a hospitalization. In recent years the model has been refined and expanded. Read, Perry, Moskowitz, and Connolly (2001), studying the etiology of schizophrenia, suggest that early traumatic stress could affect the functional biology of the developing brain thus making early stressors a contributor to the vulnerability portion of the equation. Mueser, Rosenberg, Goodman, and Trumbetta (2002) have identified a high level of co-existence of serious mental illness and PTSD and conclude that PTSD influences psychiatric disorders directly leading to avoidance, hyper-arousal, and re-experiencing of traumatic events, and in terms of its correlates of re-traumatization, substance abuse, and relationship difficulties. The model has recently been applied to depression (Hankin & Abramson, 2001), and borderline personality disorders (Zelkowitz, Paris, Guzder, & Feldman, 2001).

This model suggests that a huge, uncontrollable tragedy such as the September 11th attacks would have a major impact on our already impaired population, and that serious mental illness itself, through the mechanism of increased stress vulnerability, would be a predictor of increased risk. In the programs, therapists immediately began working to elicit their patient's responses and to help them cope with their distress. There were many anecdotal reports of patients dealing with lost family and friends, experiencing panic attacks, withdrawing and missing sessions, feeling numb and detached, and experiencing increased symptomatology. Some expressed feeling that if they had not lost someone they did not deserve to take up time. Others worried that they had somehow caused the disaster, or complained that their therapists were so caught up with providing disaster services that they, the patients, were being neglected. One case study illustrates the severe reaction of an already seriously ill patient and the members of her fragile social network.

Rosa Torres is a thirty-four year old woman of Colombian origin who is an American citizen. She is one of eleven children and lives with her mother and father, her daughter, and her profoundly retarded sister in a Manhattan apartment. The last three generations of the family have been rife with mental illness, physical abuse and neglect. Rosa's mother was neglected and abused by her mother and she in turn abused her daughter. The mother also has a psychiatric illness, and becomes bizarre and abusive when she is off of medications. Rosa was sexually abused by a family friend in adolescence, and later had several abusive relationships with husbands and boyfriends. Recently Rosa's daughter was diagnosed with a substance abuse disorder and a personality disorder and referred to a St. Luke's /Roosevelt day program.

Rosa's psychiatric problems began in early adolescence, when she saw a therapist for "shyness." Despite a substantial work history, Rosa has had ongoing psychiatric problems and been involved in various inpatient and outpatient treatment regimes. She has been variously diagnosed with schizoaffective disorder, dependent personality disorder, PTSD and panic disorder. She also has a long medical history of abdominal problems and pain involving multiple surgeries. It has been noted repeatedly that her physical condition becomes exacerbated when she is under psychological stress.

Prior to the September 11th tragedy Rosa was attending one of our day treatment programs, as a trial in our case management program had not provided the amount of structure she needed. She was doing well, and particularly benefited from a cognitively based anxiety management group run by an occupational therapist and a creative arts therapist. She found breathing exercises a particularly effective way of managing her stress and anxiety. She was focusing on beginning to develop a vocational plan.

The events of September 11th profoundly affected Rosa. One of her relatives was killed and she found herself too distraught to attend the funeral. She had an increase of panic symptoms including panic attacks and her physical condition worsened. For a week after the towers collapsed, she slept in between her parents in their bed. With continuing threats of terrorism and with the scare of anthrax, she became terrified of public transportation.

Shortly after the attacks she became too panicked to enter the subway to return home after the day program ended. Her therapist encouraged her to try the bus instead. Once on the bus Rosa's panic escalated and she heard voices telling her there was a bomb on the bus. In response to the internal voices she began screaming, "There is a bomb on the bus!" In the tense post-September 11 atmosphere, she was promptly arrested and brought to the police station. Once there, she had a bit of good luck. She explained that she was a psychiatric patient and a kind officer, finding Xeroxed directions for a breathing exercise from her anxiety reduction group in her purse, started coaching her through the exercise until she began to calm down. Her family was called and she was released to them without further incident.

That was not the end of her difficulties. In the months following the attacks Rosa's anxiety level remained high. She went to the emergency room several times for panic attacks, and was then hospitalized in a forensic unit when she was caught uncharacteristically stealing a blouse for her sister. The full impact of the September 11th tragedy and the ensuing sense of threat in the environment on Rosa and her family is still unknown. Will it be one more bump in their bumpy lives, or will it forever change the way this family copes in the city?

While many of our patients were struggling, in one way they were lucky. They enjoyed established relationships with therapists and psychiatrists trained to assist them with their reactions. Patients like Rosa were already set up with stress management and skills training groups. Yet, a group of occupational, recreational, and creative arts therapists remained concerned. We knew how difficult it was for many of our patients to develop social, functional, recreational and time management skills. We had witnessed again and again our patients' vulnerability to stress, and the resultant fearfulness, isolation, and functional decompensation. We also were experiencing ourselves the increased harshness of the changed city environment. It was impossible to avoid continual terror warnings, the war in Afghanistan, the anthrax attacks, a media focus on biological and biochemical warfare, and a challenged public transportation system. Few of us had ever faced a trauma of this magnitude. Was there a way we could offer some additional help?

The major studied psychiatric sequelae of the attacks were acute stress, PTSD and depression defined in a narrow clinical context, which we feared, could not adequately predict risk for our patients. We were unable to find data that identified role and task functioning as an outcome variable. We felt that one of the biggest threats was that the menacing environment would paralyze our patients, disrupting their functioning and inhibiting them from taking advantage of treatment, social, and recreational opportunities, shrinking their already constricted worlds even further.

The intervention we envisioned was one that would be directed at the entire outpatient population. The St. Luke's/Roosevelt programs were a major source of support for many of the patients who attended. Our hope was to use the programs to provide broadly available supports encouraging the "getting on with our normal lives" that our political leaders were advocating.

In developing a model for such a program, we were struck by an editorial by Joseph LeDoux and Jack Gorman in *The American Journal of Psychiatry* (LeDoux & Gorman, 2001). They reviewed animal studies of conditioned fear and described the anatomical pathways that lead to its development. They drew a connection between conditioned fear in rats and some of the reactions in humans subjected to overwhelming traumatic stress: withdrawal, despondence, avoidance, and intense reactions to any reminders of the event.

They continued by citing recent research showing that if rats are given a different alternative when faced with a stressful stimulus, and the stimulus stops when they make the move, they are able to utilize an "active coping model," the neurological equivalent of "getting on with life."

Translating this to human terms, LeDoux and Gorman conclude, "In practice then, the approach suggested from the laboratory studies requires that patients develop strategies that enable them to 'do something' whenever they are entertaining dysphoric thoughts or are avoiding necessary or meaningful activities. This may not be the time to encourage difficult tasks such as reading a challenging novel. Instead, the goal should simply be to successfully carry out activities, especially ones that lead to pleasure or that prevent displeasure. The rats . . . did not have to perform a difficult action–they only had to move across the chamber to succeed in ending their conditioned stimulus . . . The individual who can not bear to go back to work should be encouraged to do something else instead . . . the person might go shopping or visit a friend" (p.1955).

To the occupational therapists in the group, LeDoux and Gorman's suggestions had a familiar ring. So familiar in fact, that minus the recent research providing the scientific foundation for their remarks, their suggestions addressed an integral tenet of occupational therapy. Compare them to the remarks of Adolph Meyer (1922), addressing the Fifth Annual Meeting of the National Society for the Promotion of Occupational Therapy:

It has long been interesting to see how groups of a few excited patients can be seated in a corner in a small circle of two or three settees and kept wonderfully contented doing simple tasks not too readily arousing the desire for big movements and uncontrollable excitement, and yet not too taxing to their patience. . . A pleasure in achievement, a real pleasure in the use and activity of one's hands and muscles and a happy appreciation of time began to be used as incentives in the management of our patients.

We decided to adopt the model of active coping for our proposed intervention. We would encourage active involvement in activities that were fun, relevant, not too difficult, and had an outward focus toward socializing and engaging in the city environment. Mary Reilly, the occupational therapy theorist of the 1970s, identified this as the heart of occupational therapy, finding the "just right" activity.

We established three goals:

1. Provide and encourage access to additional social and recreational activities to psychiatric patients vulnerable to increased isolation and distress in the aftermath of September 11.
2. Reduce patient requests for increased levels of psychiatric services when the therapist assesses that the real need is for social support.
3. Support patients' return to baseline or better social and recreational functioning.

We designed a program with the working title "Reach Out and Have Some Fun" having three distinct components:

1. The Monthly Calendar: We planned to create a monthly calendar geared to our clients' needs (clear structure, easy reading level, easy availability, English and Spanish text). The calendar would list at least one free or inexpensive event a day, preferably within our catchment area, with complete information and travel directions. It would also highlight quiet and cheerful places to spend time, fun spots to bring your kids, spiritual and healing events, and ongoing activities. Because only a tiny percentage of our patients work, supporting them to get out again and hopefully to enjoy themselves would be crucial.

2. Social Coaching: We planned to provide a telephone coaching support service. Therapists who noticed signs of isolation and withdrawal in their patients could help them establish a functional goal and refer them for a social/functional coach. The coaches would be trained and professionally supervise psychology, occupational therapy, and creative arts therapy student volunteers. They would call the patients to encourage them to carry out their planned activities, invite them to report back, congratulate them upon activity completion, help them plan realistic goals, and problem solve when they had difficulty with follow-through. The telephone intervention would allow the support to be timed so that coaching reminders could take place immediately prior to the planned activity and feedback could be available immediately after. Coaches would have regular, ongoing supervision and consult with therapists as necessary. Coaching could last for up to 6 months and would focus on improving social, recreational and task functioning outside of treatment.

3. *Events:* Gatherings for all outpatients would be held at both our midtown and uptown sites either once or twice a month depending on demand and resources. The gatherings would be structured as "parties" having refreshments and a theme developed and presented by a professional occupational therapist or creative arts therapist. Examples of themes that have been suggested include the joys of pets and plants, dreams and dream catchers, starting a hobby, learning to dance the Mambo, decorating Christmas cookies, Why I love NY, and ceramic group project. Each event would include flyers advertising other events, calendars, free tickets and door prizes for those who fill out brief surveys evaluating the service. Each session would conclude with a discussion of functional "success stories" and problems. The gatherings would serve the dual goals of being pleasurable and sociable in and of themselves, and of encouraging patients to risk attending other social and recreational events not associated with the hospital.

Clients were made aware of the various goals above and were asked to select and state one with the help of their coach and record it on their referral forms (Appendix 1).

Once the program was designed, the question became how to fund it. While we were able to get started on the calendar project utilizing current staff and volunteers, the other two components required additional funding. The services we wished to provide, were not billable under the current regulations of our major payers Medicare and Medicaid. Medicare statutorily excludes any activities that are social or recreational in nature, and both payors require covered services to be provided under a doctor's treatment plan. We were defining our program as a support service rather than treatment, and wanted it to be available to the entire population. The Federal Emergency Management Agency (FEMA) funded New York State program "Project Liberty" was not a possibility either. FEMA funds were earmarked for debriefing and short term crisis counseling for individuals and groups. We were conceptualizing a program for a later stage of recovery involving longer-term intervention with services provided on an as needed basis. Near the end of 2001, we heard of the availability of funding through The Greater New York Hospital Foundation (GNYHF) Disaster Relief Fund for Crisis Counseling. This fund was set up to support the expansion of mental health, counseling and related services provided through hospitals, including the creation of new approaches to outpatient mental health services in response to community need and with an eye towards a long term recovery process. GNYHF awarded a grant to St. Luke's/Roosevelt for the project allowing for the hiring of a part time coordinator, activity specialists to run the events, and funding for the events for a one-year demonstration project.

The calendar has been distributed and the social coaching and events have begun. Though four years have passed since the buildings fell and the planes crashed, the enormity of the loss coupled with the ongoing war on terror, the continual threats of more war and more terror and the huge scar in lower Manhattan keep fear and anger alive. In a recent spirituality group run in our rehabilitation day program a discussion began about what prayers or inspirational sayings can get you through tough times. The make-up of this particular group was about 75% Hispanic patients most of whom were religious. After various group members mentioned novenas and psalms, the talk spontaneously turned to their thoughts about September 11th. How could God have let that happen they asked? How could prayer not work? One group member felt hopeful, reassuring the others that between prayer and the homeland security act no more terrorism would happen here. Another laughed nervously at this idea, saying that she heard on Spanish television that Al Qaeda members say that Americans are stupid, that they have a wide open society. One member spoke at some length about how her life had changed since September 11th. As soon as she learned the name of the man responsible for the attacks she went to an emergency room and begged them to let her kill Osama bin Laden. No one would suspect her she "reasoned." She was psychiatrically hospitalized and ever since has remained extremely nervous about going out. She, like most of the group members, is planning to stay home on the anniversary of 9/11 and pray. The therapist encouraged patients that it might help on that day to be at the program with their friends. She told them about the grant that was emphasizing return to normal activities as a way of healing, and of the first event "Latin Fiesta" that would occur in early September. They seemed excited by the idea.

While the support program has not been designed as a research study, we are making every effort to measure its efficacy. One broad measure is the degree to which it is utilized by the patients it is intended for. The calendars have been much appreciated. They are placed in the waiting area of each clinic at the beginning of the month. We regularly receive calls from the patient service representatives that the calendars have run out and need to be replaced. Staff members have asked for copies of the calendar to encourage their patients to attend events and for their own use. Quite a few patients have called us directly asking for the calendar or additional event suggestions. Others have reported sharing the calendar with friends, religious groups, and members of 12-Step programs. We hope to begin sharing the calendar with other hospital outpatient departments.

The social coaching began on September 1, 2002. In addition to measuring referrals and completed contacts, we plan to measure goals established, and goals met. Because the coaching is designed to help the patient set realistic and doable goals, our target is that 75% of the goals established will be met.

To maintain the social and festive tone of the events, we were hesitant to require outcome or satisfaction surveys. We finally settled on short survey cards, with a door prize to be given to each attendee who chooses to fill one out. In addition to attendance, we hope to gather data on some of the following questions:

1. Was the activity fun?
2. How much stress/nervousness did you feel before you came?
3. How much do you feel now?
4. Besides this activity, how many other social or recreational activities did you attend in the last week?
5. Have you ever attended any of the activities on the calendars handed out at the programs?
6. Do you have ideas for other events that you would like to see happen?
7. Did anyone encourage you to come today?

If the program should prove successful in helping patients resume or improve their level of social and recreational functioning, it will demonstrate that in non-specific ways a psychiatric outpatient program can function as a support system, mediating the impact of stress on the patients it serves. Such a service could be considered not only in response to overwhelming terrorist attacks, but as a preventive or tertiary care service in normal times. Perhaps this type of low cost, non-specifically targeted service, relying in large part on trained volunteers, can enhance the generally fragile support system of chronically ill patients, strengthening them to better endure the stresses of life. If so, we should certainly invite more of our patients to "reach out and have some fun."

ACKNOWLEDGMENTS

Thanks to Wendy Sobelman, ADTR, for providing the clinical material that is presented in this chapter, and Andrea Glasser and Jenine Klotzkin who are running the project. Names and details have been changed to protect the confidentiality of those involved.

This project is funded by a grant from the Greater New York Hospital Foundation Disaster Relief Fund.

REFERENCES

American Psychiatric Association. (1980). *Diagnostic and statistical manual of mental disorders* (3rd ed.). Washington, DC: Author.

Baker, F., Burns, T. F., Libby, M., & Intagliata, J. (1985). The impact of life events on chronic mental patients. *Hospital and Community Psychiatry, 36*(3), 299-301.

Galea, S., Ahern, J., Resnick, H., Kilpatrick, D., Bucuvalas, M., Gold, J. et al. (2002). Psychological sequelae of the September 11 terrorist attacks in New York City. *New England Journal of Medicine, 346*(13), 982-987.

Gordon, R. E., Vijay, J., Sloate, S. G., Burket, R., & Gordon, K. K. (1985). Aggravating stress and functional level as predictors of length of psychiatric hospitalization. *Hospital and Community Psychiatry, 36*(7), 773-774.

Hankin, B. L., & Abramson, L. Y. (2001). Development of gender differences in depression: An elaborated cognitive vulnerability-transactional stress theory. *Psychological Bulletin, 127*(6), 773-796.

LeDoux, J. E., & Gorman, J. M. (2001). A call to action: Overcoming anxiety through active coping. *American Journal of Psychiatry, 158*(12), 1953-1955.

Maes, M., Mylle, J., Delmeire, L., & Janca, A. (2001). Pre- and post-disaster negative life events in relation to the incidence and severity of post-traumatic stress disorder. *Psychiatry Research, 105*(1-2), 1-12.

Meyer, A. (1922). The philosophy of occupational therapy. *Archives of Occupational Therapy, 1*(1), 1-10.

Mueser, K. T., Rosenberg, S. D., Goodman, L. A., & Trumbetta, S. L. (2002). Trauma, PTSD, and the course of severe mental illness: An interactive model. *Schizophrenia Research, 53*(1-2), 123-143.

Pfefferbaum, B., Call, J. A., Lensgraf, S. J., Miller, P. D., Flynn, B. W., Doughty, D. E. et al. (2001). Traumatic grief in a convenience sample of victims seeking support services after a terrorist incident. *Annals of Clinical Psychiatry, 13*(1), 19-24.

Read, J., Perry, B. D., Moskowitz, A., & Connolly, J. (2001). The contribution of early traumatic events to schizophrenia in some patients: A traumagenic neurodevelopmental model. *Psychiatry, 64*(4), 319-345.

Schuster, M. A., Stein, B. D., Jaycox, L., Collins, R. L., Marshall, G. N., Elliott, M. N. et al. (2001). A national survey of stress reactions after the September 11, 2001, terrorist attacks. *New England Journal of Medicine, 345*(20), 1507-1512.

Smith, D. W., Christiansen, E. H., Vincent, R., & Hann, N. E. (1999). Population effects of the bombing of Oklahoma City. *Journal of Oklahoma State Medical Association, 92*(4), 193-198.

Tucker, P., Pfefferbaum, B., Nixon, S. J., & Dickson, W. (2000). Predictors of posttraumatic stress symptoms in Oklahoma City: Exposure, social support, peri-traumatic responses. *Journal of Behavioral Health Service Research, 27*(4), 406-416.

Zelkowitz, P., Paris, J., Guzder, J., & Feldman, R. (2001). Diatheses and stressors in borderline pathology of childhood: The role of neuropsychological risk and trauma. *Journal of the American Academy of Child and Adolescent Psychiatry, 40*(1), 100-105.

APPENDIX 1

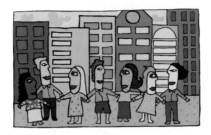

Need help getting started?

If you need some help during the week to get out to do errands, visiting, or other daily activities, take advantage of our telephone coaching program .

♦ You will receive calls to support you in getting out and/or to discuss how an activity went.

♦ You and your coach will decide a call schedule that is most helpful to you.

♦ If indicated your coach will give feedback to your therapist about how things are going.

Name:_____

Goal:_____

Phone Number:_____

Best Times to Reach: _____

_____

Therapist Signature:_____

PHOTO 1. "Art Is. . . Healing" Poster Hanging in a New York City Subway Station. Client: School of Visual Arts. Creative Director: Silas H. Rhodes. Art & Concept: Kevin O'Callaghan. Art Direction & Design: Mike Joyce & Platinum Design, Inc. NYC. Photographer: Hugh Kretschmer.

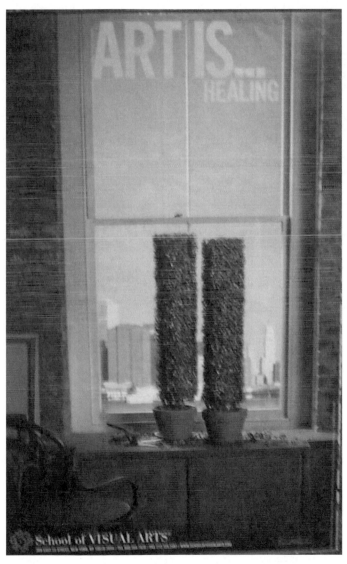

Photo by Pat Precin. Used by permission.

PART II: CREATIVITY

Creative Healing
Through Artistic Symbols

Pat Precin, MS, OTR/L

"Art is. . . Healing" is the message that Kevin O'Callaghan sends on a poster (Photo 1) he created that appeared in subway stations throughout New York City post 9/11 as part of the School of Visual Arts' subway designs, an initiative to bring artwork to subways. The window horticulture has been trimmed in the shape of the Towers and is positioned against a view of the city where the Twin Towers used to stand. Green symbolizing growth, prosperity, new life, and regeneration. Clipping shears left on the window ledge emphasize the importance of doing, re-creating and purposeful action. The view from this window is positive. Art heals.

Many other types of art including music, books, photographs, memorials, and other forms of self-expressions were created and performed by people in order to heal themselves and others and to pay tribute to the people who selflessly gave their lives to help. Handmade/community made gifts (symbols of love, strength, perseverance, hope, support,

[Haworth co-indexing entry note]: "Creative Healing Through Artistic Symbols." Precin, Pat. Co-published simultaneously in *Occupational Therapy in Mental Health* (The Haworth Press, Inc.) Vol. 21, No. 3/4, 2006, pp. 147-175; and: *Healing 9/11: Creative Programming by Occupational Therapists* (ed: Pat Precin) The Haworth Press, Inc., 2006, pp. 147-175. Single or multiple copies of this article are available for a fee from The Haworth Document Delivery Service [1-800- HAWORTH, 9:00 a.m. - 5:00 p.m. (EST). E-mail address: docdelivery@haworthpress.com].

Available online at http://www.haworthpress.com/web/OTMH
doi:10.1300/J004v21n03_10

freedom, and life) were given and received. For a year following the disaster, people became like occupational therapists, engaging in purposeful activities using expressive artistic media to get in touch with and express their feelings, and strengthen their bonds between family, friends, community and life. This chapter presents such works of art.

"Peace," written in the ashes of 9/11 with the fingertip of a survivor (Photo 2). These are ashes of human remains and of a productive society. The act of writing "Peace"; is it a desperate plea or a poignant attempt to create meaning from destruction?

A glamorous billboard advertisement remains on a building across from the previous location of the Twin Towers (Photo 3). The model trapped in Plexiglas looks as if she watched them fall. What is real? What is important? What is permanent?

Workers positioned steel beams, remnants of the World Trade Center (WTC), into the shape of a cross and erected this sculpture in the middle of Ground Zero (Photo 4) where it is easily visible from all directions. Perhaps this is an example of what Naomi Greenberg meant by her term "spiritual spontaneity" (Greenberg, 2003).

Jersey City, New Jersey, was the relief center for the rescue workers of the WTC. Survivors were to be taken here and brought to local hospitals. A strikingly graphic sculpture was erected in Jersey City (Photo 5) in memory of that horrible day, 9/11/01, on which people were fleeing out of the Towers and trying to escape falling debris. The sculpture shows a steel shard stabbing a person in the back as the person attempts to run towards safety. The Jersey City buildings in the background help recreate the scene as it occurred almost a year ago in New York City.

In 1971, Fritz Koening, commissioned by the Port Authority of New York and New Jersey, created a sculpture called "The Sphere" out of steel and bronze as a monument to world peace through trade. The 25-foot-tall Sphere, weighing 45,000 pounds, was placed on a granite fountain that once resided in the Austin J. Tobin Plaza of the WTC. On September 11, 2001, the Sphere was gashed through its center but was otherwise intact. It was removed from Ground Zero and placed in Battery Park (Photo 6) (one of the few public treasures recovered from the site) where it was unveiled on 3/11/02 by Mayor Michael Bloomberg, Gov. George Pataki, the Lower Manhattan Development Corporation, and former Mayor Rudolph Giuliani as a memorial to people who lost their lives at the WTC. The Sphere has endured the tragedy and now stands as a symbol of resilience, strength and hope. Upon viewing it in March of 2002, its creator, Fritz Koening, stated that it now has its own life–a beauty that it did not originally possess.

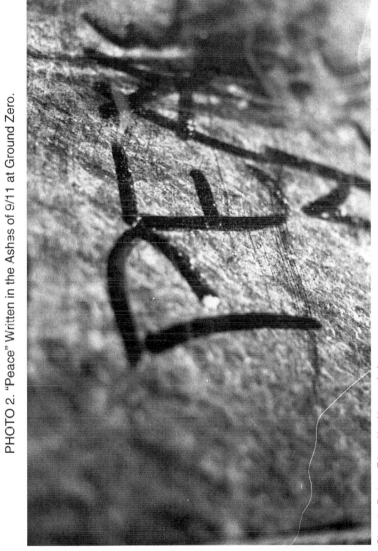

PHOTO 2. "Peace" Written in the Ashes of 9/11 at Ground Zero.

Photo by Barbara Ethan. Used by permission.

PHOTO 3. A Storefront Advertisement Remains on a Building Across the Street from Ground Zero.

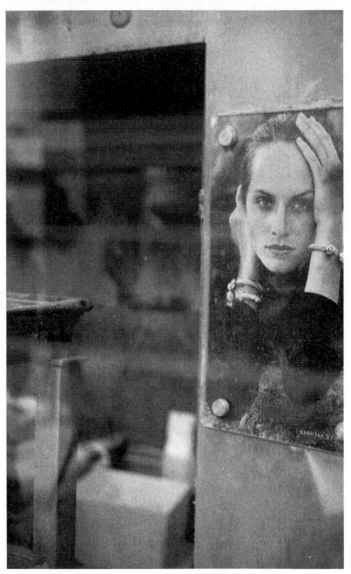

Photo by Barbara Ethan. Used by permission.

PHOTO 4. A Cross Made of Steel Beams from the World Trade Center Set in Concrete at the Site of Ground Zero Can Be Seen in All Directions.

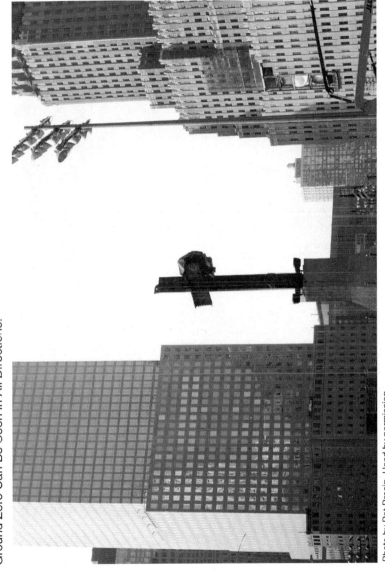

PHOTO 5. A Memorial Sculpture in Jersey City. A Steel Shard from the WTC Penetrates a Fleeing Person.

PHOTO 6. The Sphere: A Sculpture that Survived the Disaster, Now a Symbol of Resilience, Strength and Hope in its New Home, Battery Park. Sculpture by Fritz Koening, 1971.

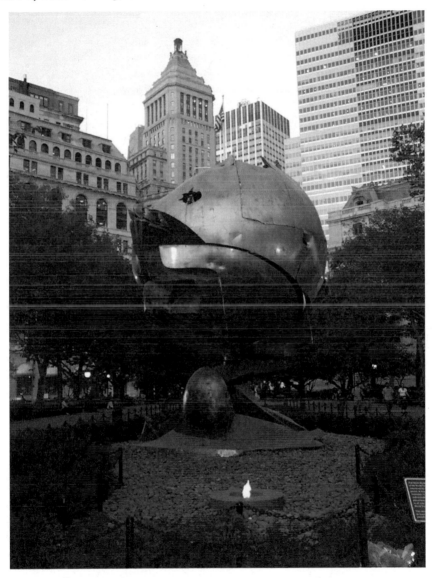

Photo by Pat Precin. Used by permission.

The Tribute in Light was created to honor and remember people who died in the 9/11 attack on the WTC. The Municipal Art Society collaborated with other civic organizations and a team of multidisciplinary artists to create two columns of 44 spotlights whose beams projected for a mile into the city sky from a site near Ground Zero. These beams powered by 7,000-watt xenon bulbs focused two rays that resembled the WTC Towers. They were said to have equaled the power of two million light bulbs and could be seen for up to 25 miles in any direction under optimal conditions. On the sixth month anniversary of the disaster, 3/11/02, Mayor Michael Bloomberg and Gov. George Pataki of New York dedicated the Tribute in Light to people lost at Ground Zero and to the city's strength and renewal. The lighting of the Tribute in Light was one of multiple dedications that took place throughout the United States on 3/11/02. Its beams stood as pillars of strength for 32 days from dusk to 11 p.m., a symbol of hope to families of lost ones, New Yorkers and the world.

Following 9/11, members of the Refuse and Resist! Artists' Network talked to other artists about what had happened, how they felt about it, and what may happen in the future. They, along with other artists developed a powerful performance piece, "OUR GRIEF IS NOT A CRY FOR WAR." They held performances in Time Square and in Union Square where over 175 artists stood silently for an hour in a straight line formation, wearing black clothes and dust masks and carrying signs that read, "Our Grief is not a Cry for War" (Photo 7).

"Liberty George" Dukov was born in 1944 in Bulgaria where he studied structural design (also at the Academy of Art in Holle, Germany). He came to New York in 1991 in search of a "free spirit" in his artwork and created his first mask. Since 9/11, Liberty George has been designing masks that relate to the terrorist attacks on America. His Statue of Liberty series includes masks in the shape of the head of the real Statue of Liberty (Photo 8).

One such mask has the photographs on it of all 343 firefighters who died at the World Trade Center on it. Liberty George stated that "all 343 pictures fit perfectly." "Never before has this happened. I don't measure, just with eye, it may be a spirit, but they fit." Liberty George's father died in 1999. He had been a famous sculptor. Liberty George feels that his father left him the "spirit of creativity" through which he can realize his American dream. He does not have his green card, but immigration has approved his stay in the U.S. on a yearly basis. For this, he is grateful. In return, he creates masks containing the "American spirit."

Another of his masks is comprised of the 37 Port Authority Police who died in the disaster. The caption on the mask reads, "We salute

PHOTO 7. "OUR GRIEF IS NOT A CRY FOR WAR" Performance Piece in Union Square Park Performed by Refuse & Resist! Artists' Network.

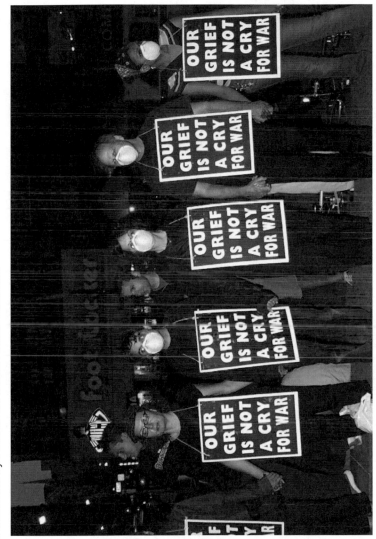

Photo by Pat Precin. Used by permission.

PHOTO 8. Liberty Masks for Sale in Union Square Park by "Liberty George" Dukov.

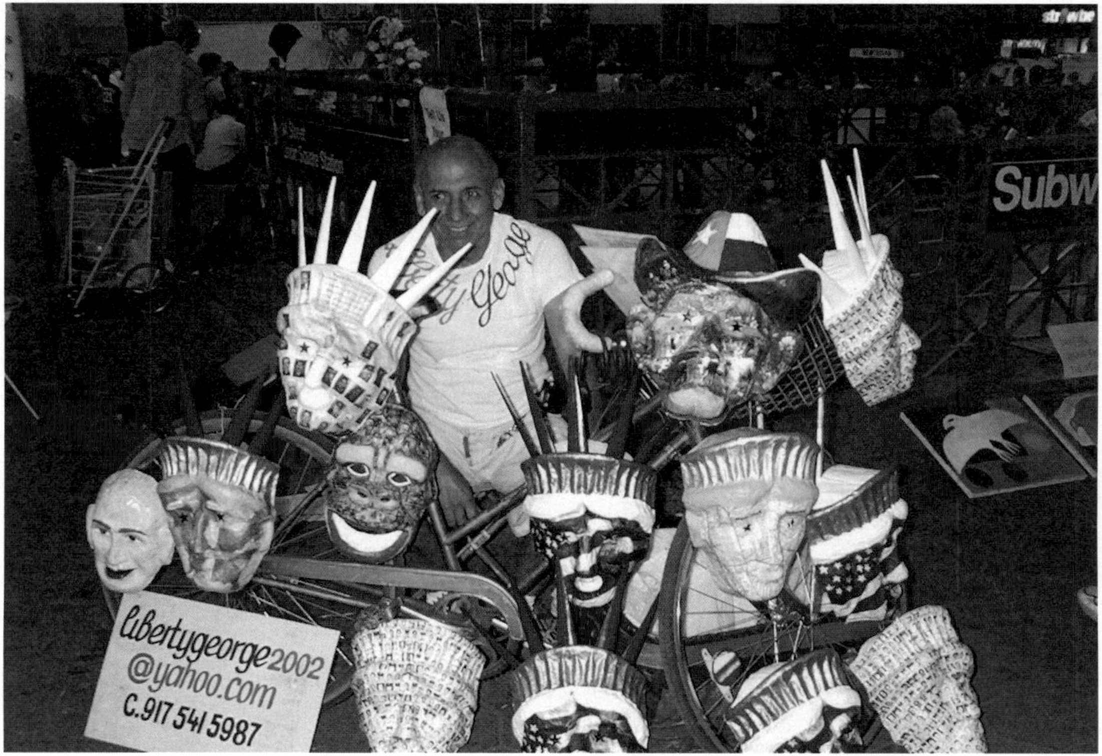

these 37 Heroes from the Port Authority Police Department on September 11, 2001. These officers along with their courageous brothers and sisters aided thousands of employees and visitors caught in the WTC attacks. Their courageous efforts exemplify the Port Authority Police Department's commitment to serve and protect the public. God bless."

Liberty George states that his third Statue of Liberty mask, "Lady Liberty," is his most powerful. With an eagle on the crown of her head and the eagle's wings swooping across her face in the colors of the American flag, it too contains the American spirit of freedom that "even the terrorists cannot kill because I put the spirit in her face forever." "This mask was born in Astoria [Queens, New York] in a basement in the darkness," Liberty George relays. "When I put my mind to something, I do it, and making these masks takes my mind off of my problems."

Liberty George's masks are in collections in Tokyo, Berlin, Sydney, Paris, Switzerland, Madrid, Milan and in New York (the Pratt Institute, the Folk Art Museum Shop, the Norman Schaffer Gallery, An American Craftsman, Adrian Van der Plas Pier 17, and the Williamsburg Art and Historical Center), but his favorite place to show his art is on the Queensboro Bridge as biking weather permits.

Another New York artist, Slink Moss, created a series of soaring birds (oil on canvas) entitled, "Phoenix Rising from the Ashes. . ." (Photo 9) displayed in front of a New York City subway station. The phoenix is a cross-cultural mythical bird of extreme beauty with scarlet and gold plumage and a melodious cry. Each phoenix lived for at least 500 years, but only one existed at any given time. When the phoenix felt old, it made a mortuary nest of aromatic wood, cinnamon, spikenard and myrrh in a sacred tree. The heat of the rising sun set its nest on fire, and the phoenix burned to a pile of silver-grey ash. Three days later, the ashes shook and from them came a newborn phoenix to live another 500 years. The ancient Egyptians believed that the phoenix stood for immortality. Clement of Rome was the first Christian (near the end of the first century) to believe that the myth symbolized the resurrection and life after death. In Japanese culture, it represents capacity for vision, intense excitement and deathless inspiration. In Chinese mythology, it is the symbol of prosperity, power, grace and high virtue. In Slink Moss' creations, the birds depict hope rising out of the terrorists' destruction.

Buildings in New York City became popular canvases for artwork. Their tall, massive structures lend themselves well to sending messages such as the one in Photo 10, "The human spirit is not measured by the size of the act, but by the size of the heart." The "heart" in this instance is some 50 stories high.

PHOTO 9. "Phoenix Rising from the Ashes" Oil on Canvas Created and Displayed by Artist Slink Moss at the Entrance to a New York City Subway.

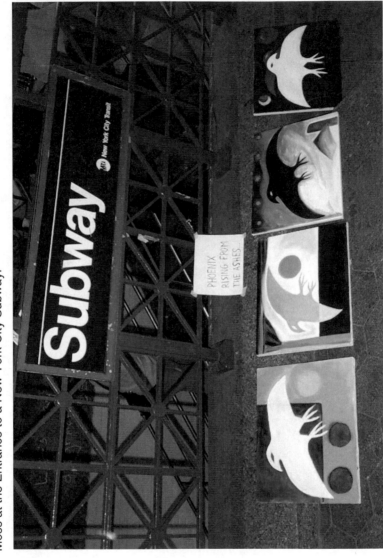

PHOTO 10. A Building Near Ground Zero Hosts a Mural Tribute to the Human Spirit.

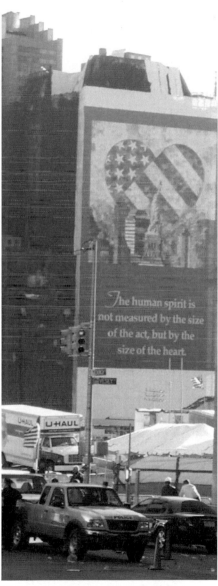

Photo by Pat Precin. Used by permission.

On a smaller scale, the World Trade Center buildings have been shrunk and encapsulated in the shatterproof glass of a liquid globe as shown in Photo 11. This safe, womb-like environment shows a perfect city, impenetrable from the outside.

"Chambers Street Station, World Trade Center," the subway stop of many after 9/11 (Photo 12). What did they see on their way to Ground Zero? What did they leave? Hats, underwear, posters, flags, banners, and T-shirts, lining fences with messages of terrorist termination, peace, love, sorrow, prayer, unity, and revenge (Photos 13-16). Adhering to another wall near Ground Zero is an array of patches that had been worn by firefighters and police who died in the disaster (Photo 17). Farther down is a chain memorial in the shape of a cross under which people have left tokens of coins, religious figures, hair pins and other things on their person as they walk by (Photo 18). The inscription beneath the cross reads, "9/11/01. This Cross, Once a Chain, Was Found by a Fireman Digging in the Rubble for Those Who Were Lost. May All Those Who Perished Rest in Peace. John Misha, FDNY Ground Zero."

Union Square Park located at 14th Street in Manhattan became a gathering place for people to express themselves. People engaged in chalk drawings (Photo 19) by day and candle lighting rituals by night (Photo 20). The Empire State Building lit up in red, white and blue can be seen in the background of a Union Square gathering (Photo 21) on the first year anniversary, 9/11/02.

Fran Babiss, an occupational therapist from New York City who found herself in France on 9/11/01, created a collage of the Tower ruins juxtaposed with the town in France (Rogny) where she made a silent tribute (Photo 22). Creating this collage helped her psychologically bring the events of New York to her location in Rogny where she was then able to mourn on September 14, 2001 at 12 Noon.

Many handmade/community made gifts from around the world were sent to New York as gestures of hope. A sculpture of a bear came from Germany with painted symbols of patriotism, the spiral of life, longevity, and symbols to ward off evil (Photo 23). The bear stands just outside of Bowling Green Park in lower Manhattan with a plaque beneath that reads, "This Buddy Bear is a gift of the City of Berlin to New York, symbolizing the friendship of the people living in the two cities. It was painted by the Berlin artist Helge Leiberg and presented to the City of New York on May 7, 2002."

A gift of 1,000 cranes was given by Bow High School students and hangs in front of a church near Ground Zero (Photo 24). The thousand cranes are a symbol of peace and come from a story about a young girl,

PHOTO 11. A "Snow Globe" of the WTC.

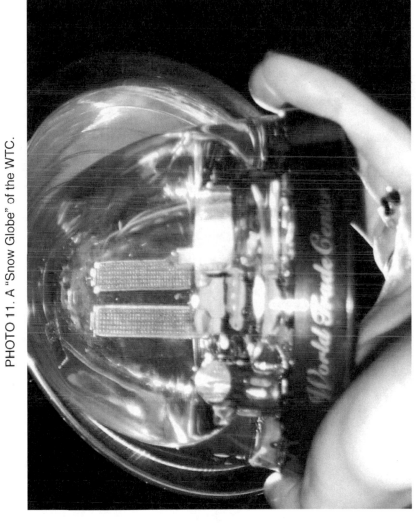

Photo by Pat Precin. Used by permission.

PHOTO 12. Chambers Street Subway Station—a Popular Stop for Ground-Zero Visitors.

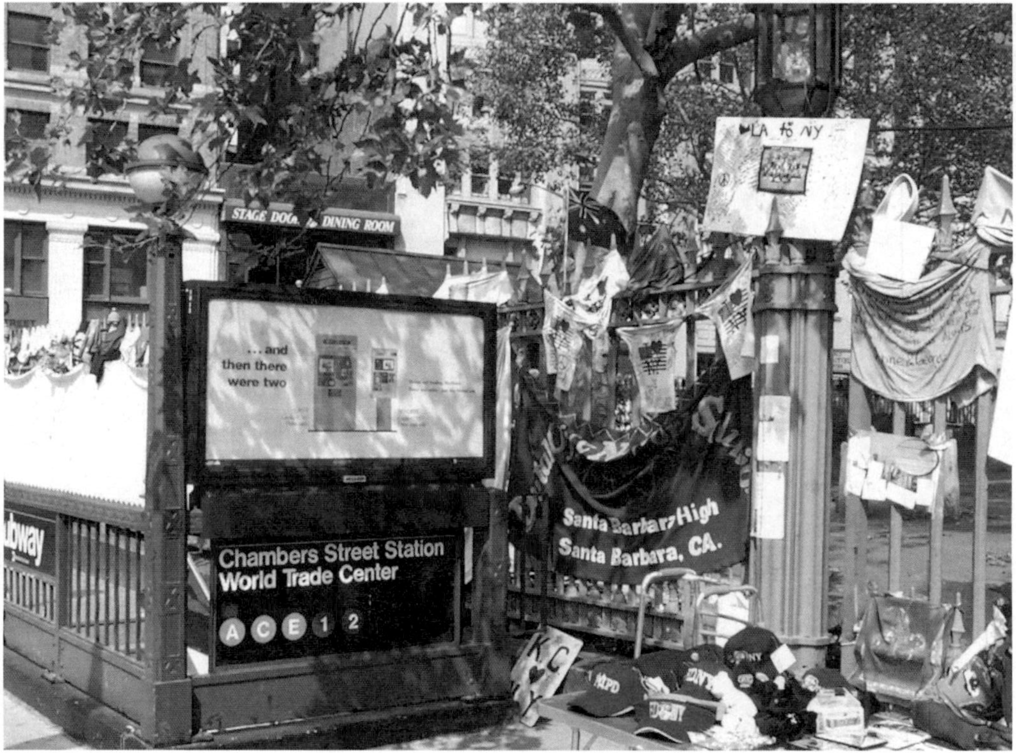

Photo by Pat Precin. Used by permission.

PHOTO 13. Hats Off to the Heroes.

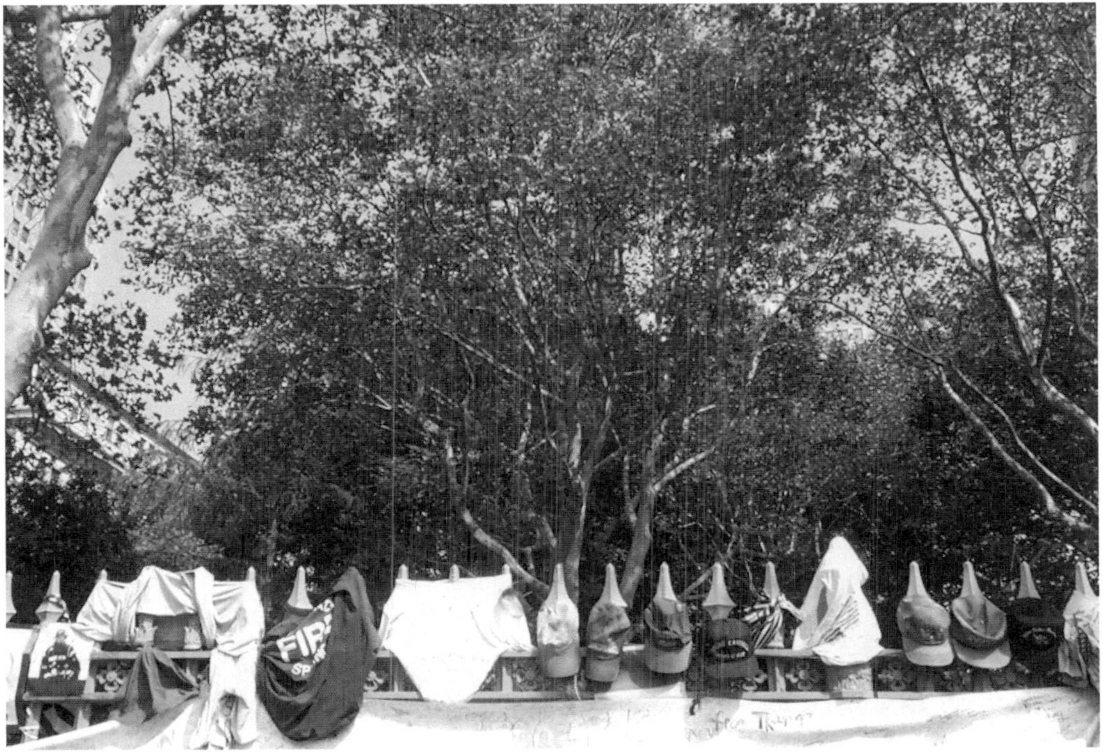

Photo by Pat Precin. Used by permission.

PHOTO 14. Memorabilia Left by People From All Over the World on a Fence Near Ground Zero.

Photo by Pat Precin. Used by permission.

PHOTO 15. T-shirts, Flags, Hats, Posters, and Banners with Messages that Range from Revenge to Peace.

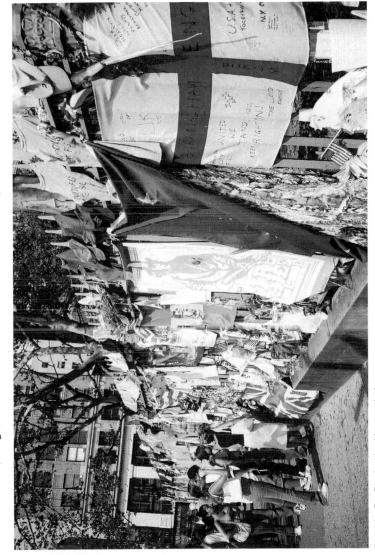

PHOTO 16. A Message to Terminate the Terrorists.

PHOTO 17. An Array of Police and Firefighters' Patches Whose Owners Are No Longer Alive.

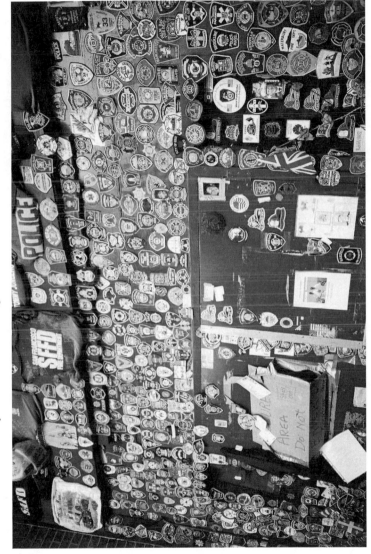

Photo by Pat Precin. Used by permission.

PHOTO 18. A Chain Memorial in the Shape of a Cross Displayed Near Ground Zero.

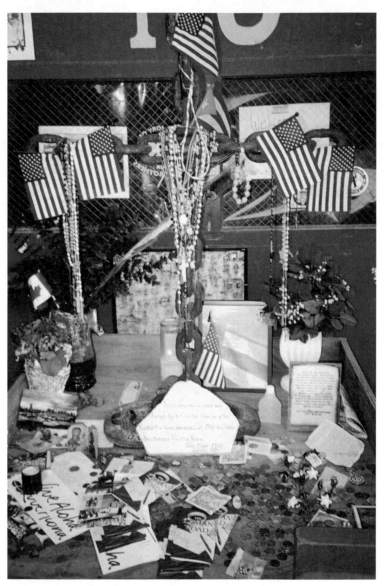

Photo by Pat Precin. Used by permission.

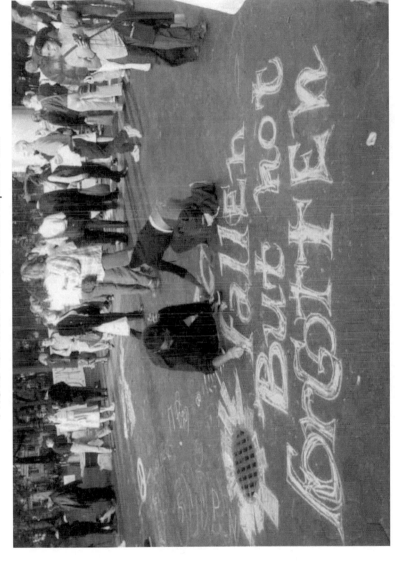

PHOTO 19. Artists at Work in Union Square Park.

Photo by Fran Babiss. Used by permission.

PHOTO 20. Three Girls Are Lighting Red, White, and Blue Candles on the First Anniversary, 9/11/02.

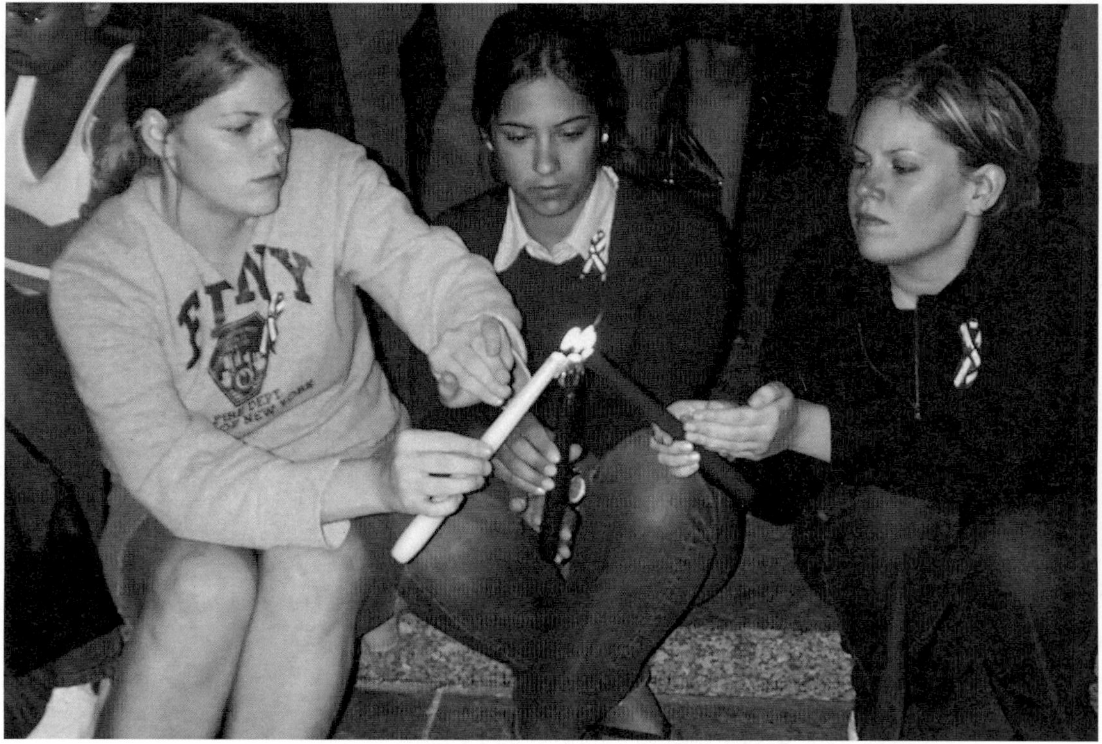

Photo by Pat Precin. Used by permission.

PHOTO 21. A Red, White, and Blue Empire State Building in the Background of an Evening Anniversary Gathering in Union Square Park, 9/11/02.

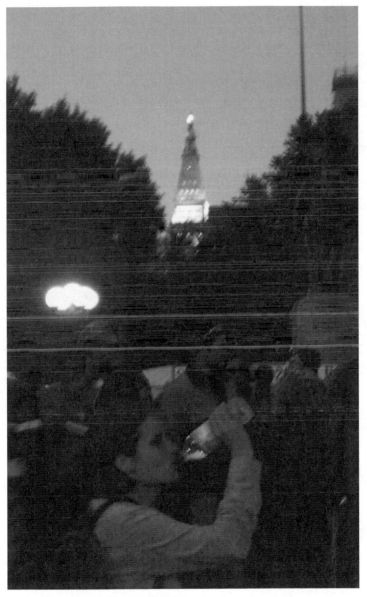

Photo by Pat Precin. Used by permission.

PHOTO 22. A Collage of Remnants of the WTD Superimposed in the City of Rogny, France.

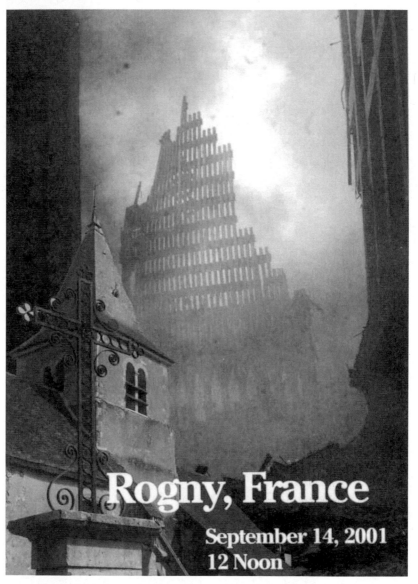

Photo by Fran Babiss. Used by permission.

PHOTO 23. The Buddy Bear. A Gift from Germany Painted by the Berlin Artist, Helge Leiberg, Stands Near Bowling Green Park.

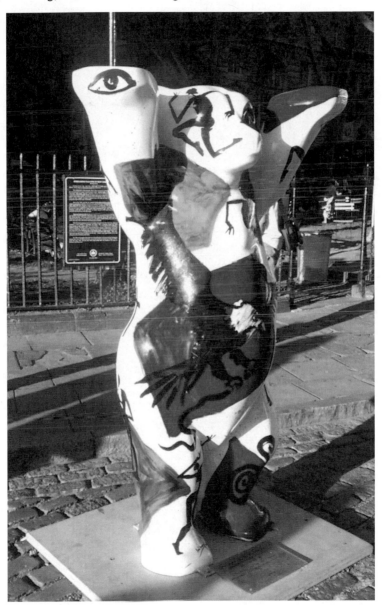

Photo by Pat Precin. Used by permission.

PHOTO 24. Gift of a Thousand Cranes Created by Bow High School Students.

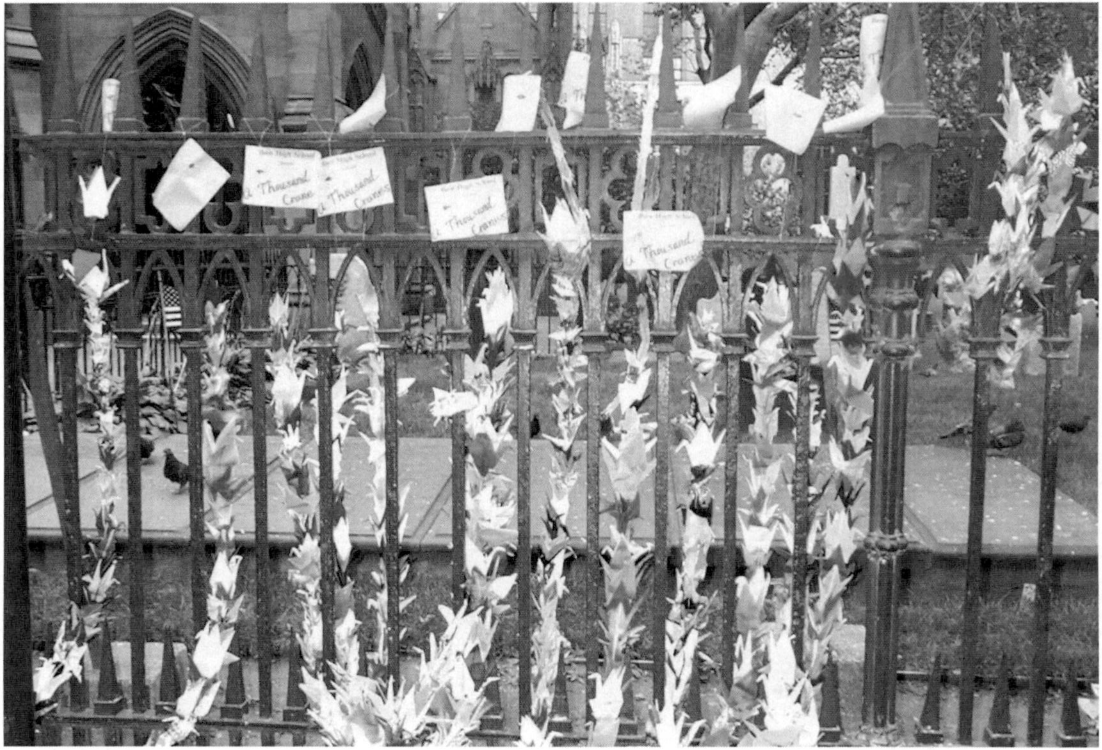

Photo by Pat Precin. Used by permission.

Satchi, who suffered from radiation sickness after the bombing of Hiroshima. To keep her mind occupied, her mother told her that if she could fold a thousand cranes out of her medicine wrappers, she would be well again. She died before finishing all one thousand, but her friends finished them for her.

Widows of the disaster who gave birth after September 11 were inspired to send a message of healing. They made a necklace of over 10,000 Band-Aids. Each Band-Aid (donated by Wal-Mart and Johnson & Johnson) carried a message of hope from the Orange County community of California. The necklace was laid around Ground Zero on Memorial Day of 2002 by Michelle Parent, a 12-year-old from Lake Forest, California. In Chicago, a giant rope was woven from residents' personal belongings that were near and dear to their hearts. The rope consisted of military uniforms, wedding dresses, graduation gowns, and baby blankets, all transitional objects full of memories that stretched the length of a football field. The rope was given to the firefighters of New York City as a symbol of hope. David Xui, an artist from Canada, having lost a friend in the attacks, painted portraits on eggshells of the 343 firefighters who lost their lives and offered them as gifts.

In the chapters to follow, an occupational therapy student describes the therapeutic benefits of a flag pin project (chapter by Janine Gallo) while Jeanne Lewin brings to consciousness the dark side of creativity in her chapter entitled, "The Unspoken Words: Reflections on a Keynote Address Following 9/11."

REFERENCE

Greenberg, N. (2003). Spiritual spontaneity: Developing our own 9/11: One Occupational Therapist's spiritual journey across the 9/11 divide. In P. Precin (Ed.), *Surviving 9/11: Impact and Experiences of Occupational Therapy Practitioners* (pp. 153-189). New York: Haworth Press.

BIBLIOGRAPHY

Liberty George Dukov, Accessed September 10, 2002 from libertygeorge2000@hotmail.com.
Refuse and Resist!, Accessed September 10, 2002 from http://www.refuseandresist.org.
School of Visual Arts, Accessed September 10, 2002 from http://www.schoolofvisualarts.edu.

Pinning the Pieces Back Together. . .

Janine Gallo, BA, OTS

I distinctly remember situating myself on the express bus early morning on September 11, 2001. I set my bag on the floor, reclined my seat, and closed my eyes to take advantage of the extra forty-five minute rest I was afforded. As usual, I woke up at West 4th and Waverly Place, exited the bus, and began what I believed would be a routine day of graduate classes at New York University. Little did I know that after stepping foot off that bus my life and the lives of Americans would be changed forever. The events that followed during that day will be etched in my memory for an eternity.

After our first class, three of my friends and I took a walk to a local copy shop to pick up one of the many packets of required readings we needed for the fall semester. As we walked, we laughed and joked about the slim chance that our next class would be canceled. Little did we know the irony of our complaints. We purchased our packets and left the copy shop to reluctantly head to class. Just as we stepped out the door, a man approached us and said that a plane had just hit the World Trade Center. Initially we dismissed him as "just another crazy New Yorker," until we looked up and saw the evidence of his words.

As my friends and I gazed up at the skyline, we were astonished to see a gaping hole in the side of the Twin Towers, spewing out smoke. At that moment, all my sheltered and protected mind could ascertain was that it was some sort of fancy movie stunt that would trick us all into be-

[Haworth co-indexing entry note]: "Pinning the Pieces Back Together. . . ." Gallo, Janine. Co-published simultaneously in *Occupational Therapy in Mental Health* (The Haworth Press, Inc.) Vol. 21, No. 3/4, 2006, pp. 177-182; and: *Healing 9/11: Creative Programming by Occupational Therapists* (ed: Pat Precin) The Haworth Press, Inc., 2006, pp. 177-182. Single or multiple copies of this article are available for a fee from The Haworth Document Delivery Service [1-800- HAWORTH, 9:00 a.m. - 5:00 p.m. (EST). E-mail address: docdelivery@haworthpress.com].

Available online at http://www.haworthpress.com/web/OTMH
doi:10.1300/J004v21n03_11

lieving that a terrible accident had just occurred. In my denial-ridden mind, we were experiencing another "War of the Worlds" phenomenon. Convinced that there was no need to worry, we continued on to our next class.

As we walked, I exchanged glances with many people passing by; these were glances I will never erase from my mind. They were looks of sadness, fear, and bewilderment. It did not take long for my friends and I to adopt such emotions. Our pace quickened, and when we arrived at our class, we were met with tears, panic, and looks of horror. These feelings quickly invaded my body and before I knew it I was crying and shaking, searching for some sense of security. My classmates all cried together, embraced, and frantically scurried around trying to reach loved ones for some feeling of normalcy, but to no avail. None of our cell phones were working and the land lines were switching on and off. We were stuck and frozen with fear, hearing only the blaring sounds of sirens in the distance and weeping everywhere.

We stared into one another's eyes feeling so helpless and idle. The only emotion I did not feel at that time was loneliness. I knew one thing for certain. We had one another. We stayed together all morning. We watched the first tower fall in disbelief, and were left speechless as we witnessed the second tower plunge to the ground. Each one of us took turns breaking down as others stepped forward to console. As the day progressed, our class dwindled in numbers. People began to scatter all over the city, searching for a safe place to spend the night. We parted ways with loving words and fearful good-byes, wondering what would happen next. . .

Classes were cancelled for the next few days because everything south of 14th Street was closed. Our city was shut down. . . no one allowed in and no one allowed out. Threats of future attacks were reported one after the other on the television and radio and in newspapers and magazines. Americans everywhere were scared. . . scared to even leave their homes. My classmates and I sat cooped up in our homes making endless phone calls trying to make some sense out of complete chaos. We spoke with one another about how we felt so powerless and helpless. We all called our local fire departments, police departments, Red Crosses, and Salvation Armies. None of them needed any more volunteers. There were no survivors to help. All they needed now was money.

Being graduate students at New York University, none of us could afford to simply write out a large check. One thing we could donate was our time, but no one needed volunteers. What could we do to help? I knew that taking a collection would not ease our feelings of despair. It simply would not be enough.

A friend reminded me of flag pins we used to make as children out of safety pins and tiny red, white, and blue seed beads. I thought that as a class we could make these pins as well as some red, white and, blue ribbons to sell. When classes resumed, I presented the idea to the first and second year occupational therapy students. My fellow classmates agreed that it was a good idea and decided to meet as a group in between classes to assemble them.

As we sat tediously stringing each bead onto the pins, an amazing change came about. We all started sharing our feelings with one another. With each bead we threaded, a new story was told or a new fear was discovered. Our psyches in essence were linking together forming a beautiful picture that told each of our stories in a separate yet cohesive way, just as each individual safety pin linked together to form a unified flag. We talked about the future, what was in store for us, and how fortunate we were to be there. We joked and managed to forget the task at hand and become immersed in one another. We learned a lot about each other in those hours and I feel that these meetings became a psychological outlet for all of us. It was a safe time to feel selfless and giving, something we all needed to internalize at that time.

We discussed how this was the first disaster that our generation had to face, and conjectured as to how we felt our peers and ourselves would cope with such tragedy. We pondered the idea that we would be revisited by this horror not only in our personal lives, but in our professional lives as well. Because of this, we realized that we needed to come to terms with this catastrophe. I believe that simply by coming together in a group, focused on one goal, we started this ongoing "recovery" process. We established a strong support network that not only helped us to cope, but also has since expanded to become great friendships and wonderful professional resources.

And the pins sold themselves. Everyone was asking for them, and it was hard to keep up with the demand. People wore them everyday, for months afterward. At the end of our fall semester we tallied up our profits and were proud to discover that we had raised $1,400. This may not seem like a large sum, however, to us it represented more than just money. It was a concrete result of hours of caring and concern we offered. It made us feel as though we served a purpose by helping our country to recover and survive.

We met one last time to decide to whom we would donate the profits. We had many options to choose from, charity organizations seemed to be popping up everywhere. Our options spanned from personally adopting a family to donating the money to the American Red Cross. After much research and deliberation, we agreed to donate the money to the Twin Tower Fund, which was established by former Mayor Rudolph Guliani. We felt it was a reputable charity and we knew our money would definitely go to help the families of the World Trade Center victims.

I composed a short letter (see Appendix) and bought a greeting card for us all to sign to send in with our donation. I wanted my classmates to have the opportunity to sign their names and finalize the project we had worked so hard to bring about. I also wanted us to be able to establish closure. This is not to say that I felt we should forget all that had happened, but I wanted us to be able to look back and feel as though we started something, followed through with it, finished it, and were able to move on. We could have continued fund-raising; but I believe we had reaped all of the benefits we could from it. We not only raised money, but also raised each other's awareness and helped each other begin to heal. We needed to make the next step in the recovery process and that step was integrating this catastrophe into our everyday lives in a functional and healthy way. We had to learn how to move on.

The pin making groups functioned as a support group for us. We established a support network that was at our disposal daily. The resulting bonds and confidences that were established helped us to feel safe to move on. We had one another to turn to. We always had someone to look to for encouragement.

Having a group to relate to and share emotions with is a fundamental principle that serves as the foundation for many Occupational Therapy frames of reference. Throughout our semesters of study at the New York University, we learned about the importance of group process and human interaction in relation to healing and coping. We were taught this in theory but never experienced this phenomenon first hand until our group meetings following September 11. These meetings served as evidence of the benefits an activity group can have with individuals experiencing trying times, whether it be mental illness, drug abuse, or in our case stress and fear. In these meetings we each filled the role of peer, leader, educator, learner, and Occupational Therapist. We experienced the emotions our future and current clients experience in the groups we will and currently do run. This type of understanding is an invaluable asset that we might never have had the opportunity to have if not for the pin-making meetings. The reward that we received from making the pins runs far deeper than merely raising money for a worthy cause. We learned to trust, to heal, to lead, to be led, when to hold on, and how to let go. . . and most importantly we learned the value of people in our lives and how much we have to offer one another simply by extending ourselves.

To say that this journey towards recovery and reestablishment of normalcy is over would be a fallacy. Each day every American carries the memory of September 11 close to their heart. My classmates and I are no different. The things we saw and the emotions we felt will never be replicated and never be erased from our minds. However, we are very fortunate because along with reliving the sadness and fear we are able to remember the support we offered one another. Now as we approach the one-year anniversary of this devastation, I have renewed faith in people and the strength and caring that they are capable of. My friends and I can look back on such a catastrophe and instead of feeling powerless and scared, we can remember that we did something to help. As a group we united not only to help our country heal but to help one another heal. This is something that I think of and am thankful for every day of my life.

APPENDIX. Letter to the World Trade Center Fund

January 30, 2002

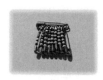 Dear Sir or Madam:

I am writing this letter representing the first and second year Occupational Therapy students at New York University.

Being so close to the September 11th disaster, we watched in shock and disbelief as the Twin Towers collapsed. We felt very helpless and scared and had few outlets for such fear and vulnerability. As a class, we decided to raise funds for the families of those tragically lost on the 11th. We made patriotic ribbons and flag pins to sell during our fall semester. We sold them, and managed to raise a total of $1,400.00 for your fund.

We would like to thank you for your efforts to help those in need and we hope that our contribution will help to make a difference.

Sincerely,

Janine Gallo,
New York University Occupational Therapy World Trade Center Fundraising Chair

The Unspoken Words:
Reflections on a Keynote Address
Following 9/11

Jeanne E. Lewin, MS, OTR/L

The events of 9/11 influenced all of us in different ways. I was not directly involved in the New York City, Washington, DC, or Pennsylvania rescue efforts nor suffered any losses of loved ones in the terrorist attacks of September 11, 2001. However, the events of that dreadful event actively influenced my role as an occupational therapist. I had been invited to give a keynote presentation November 2. The story below reflects thoughts that crossed my mind as I felt a need to incorporate the ways that the attacks on America influenced us all after 9/11. The keynote address was to be given to occupational therapists at a state fall conference.

I was thrilled and flattered to have been invited to give the keynote address to the Illinois Occupational Therapy Association's Fall Conference, November 2001. Having been the keynote speaker the previous year at the Ohio Occupational Therapy Association's 2000 Fall Conference, I felt somewhat prepared because the topics of the two keynotes were similar. *Creativity on the Edge of Possibility* was the title. The mission: to introduce tools for managing change in our professional and personal lives. With some "regional" updates and tweaks to the talk, the Illinois presentation would be similar in content to that presented in

[Haworth co-indexing entry note]: "The Unspoken Words: Reflections on a Keynote Address Following 9/11." Lewin, Jeanne E. Co-published simultaneously in *Occupational Therapy in Mental Health* (The Haworth Press, Inc.) Vol. 21, No. 3/4, 2006, pp. 183-190; and: *Healing 9/11: Creative Programming by Occupational Therapists* (ed: Pat Precin) The Haworth Press, Inc., 2006, pp. 183-190. Single or multiple copies of this article are available for a fee from The Haworth Document Delivery Service [1-800- HAWORTH, 9:00 a.m. - 5:00 p.m. (EST). E-mail address: docdelivery@haworthpress.com].

doi:10.1300/J004v21n03_12   *183*

Ohio the year before. This interactive, audience participatory session would answer the following questions: What is creativity?, What are the attributes of a creative thinker?, and What are some tools of creative thinking? To conclude the presentation, the participants would experience the creative process through a group activity. Simple. I had planned to provide an energizing presentation to engage the audience in such a way to facilitate confidence in the participants. The culminating activity would show the attendees that everyone, in some small way, is indeed creative.

The participants would leave at the end of the presentation wearing bright yellow buttons proclaiming, "I am a human becoming!" The buttons were created in the spirit that we have been human beings long enough. The green text (green to symbolize growth, creativity, and forward movement) on the buttons suggested that it is time to think of ourselves as part of a process, a metamorphosis of evolving that continues throughout the life span.

The acts of the terrorists toward the United States of America on September 11, 2001 totally changed the context in which the audience would be receiving my keynote. As a responsibility to the audience, the context necessitated that I incorporate references to the "events." But how and in what way might I bring up the events over which we were still very much in shock and disbelief? What would be the "just right" fit to keep the audience motivated to engage in an hour of experiencing creative thinking without channeling their thoughts toward the attacks, and in doing so, losing their attention to the topic of creative thinking? And even more profound, to my surprise was that the more I pondered how to incorporate the events of 9/11 into the presentation, what crystallized was the thought that what the terrorists did to America was the epitome of creative thinking! Their actions were a manifestation of the *dark side* of creative thinking!

As the November date drew closer, the incubation process of creative thinking was well under way. Like a chicken that incubates its eggs by sitting on them, a similar phenomenon happens when we are faced with a creative challenge. Somewhere back in the far reaches of our psyche what can best be called "creative tension" presents itself. Creative tension (Lewin & Reed, 1998) feels like a gap that needs to be closed. It is that which motivates us to pursue our goals and create the future. To recognize the root of the tension, we must make explicit our starting place or the present reality. Next, we define our destination. In the case of the keynote, my starting place was an already written address. The challenge, tension, or gap was caused by the events of 9/11. My destination or future state was the incorporation of the 9/11 events into the keynote.

How do we move from the present state to creating a future, one that reduces the tension? One way is by keeping an open mind and maintaining what the Brain Mind Based educators Renate and Geoffrey Caine (Caine & Caine, 1994) call a state of "relaxed alertness." As we move through the events and experiences of our daily lives, we intuitively "frame" the occurrences within the context of the challenge that we need to satisfy. To help the process along, I read and listened to everything that was within my reach about the September 11 atrocities. Then one day I found the way to segue the 9/11 incidents to creative thinking.

The October 13, 2001 *Wall Street Journal* reported a story regarding a primary grade school history book that needed to be rewritten since the September 11 attack. In a section heading on the topic of the attacks, the authors opted for the phrase "United We Stand" over "America Under Attack" in an effort to spare the emotions of their young audience. The article continued to describe another leading history book publisher who opted for the title "Our Nation Recovers." Both authors used phrases to introduce possibly one of the most negative events in the history of the USA with a phrase that had a positive ring. Creative thinkers keep moving forward (KMF) (Smith, 1997). In the spirit of creative thinking, the two historians demonstrated that framing their thoughts with positive words was more empowering to their readers than moving backwards towards negative, nonproductive thinking. The essence of creative thinking is thinking positive, moving forward. *Fine*, I thought. *This information fits into the talk and brings in the events. Why, then, was I still restless, not satisfied to KMF, and create the talk as I had planned?*

What I really wanted to describe in the keynote was the way in which the terrorists were creative in their evilness.

Talking about creative thinking in the wake of September 11 seemed sacrilegious following the events that we had each experienced. The terrorists were truly creative in what they did when they attacked the Pentagon in Washington and the World Trade Towers in New York City. They hijacked four jet planes from the would-be victims of their terrorism, the United States. They selected planes that were sure to have full fuel tanks due to their scheduled cross-country destination. And, they used them as weapons against us on our turf! This was the ultimate out-of-the-box thinking. These thoughts were clearly something that I dared not talk about in the keynote. Thinking about what happened to our country barely two months prior was painful beyond words yet so obviously the most overt, glaring example of creativity that each of us had experienced. Still I was unwilling to take the risk of presenting these thoughts in deference to protecting the audience's emotional well-being. Then again, was not risk-taking one of the key attributes of creative thinking? But so is empathy. Therein lay another quandary in my developing the presentation.

To develop one's skill or FORTE for creative thinking, one must be:

Flexible,
Open-minded,
Risk taking,
Tolerant with ambiguity, and
Empathetic or understanding for the other point of view.

To support the flexible part of the participants' thinking, I had planned to show the graphic (Figure 1) of the plane. To elicit their participation, I would ask the audience, "Is the plane coming or going? Raise your hand if you think the plane is flying *toward* you. Raise your hand if you think the plane is flying *away* from you. Now see if you can perceive the plane to move both toward and away from you?" However, how dare I show the airplane example so soon after September 11? I felt the necessity to delete the plane experience altogether.

Although I deemed that the plane example was a stronger choice for the experience that I was assimilating, I did not think it was the wisest choice with respect to the current state of events that had recently transpired. So in its place, I decided to use the book (Figure 2) instead. Similar to the questions related to the airplane example, the audience was

FIGURE 1

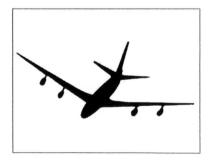

FIGURE 2

asked whether the book was facing toward or away from the viewer. Then, they were challenged to try to shift their perceptions to a perspective opposite to that of their initial impression upon viewing it.

Per the original plan in creating the presentation's content, the audience's take home message was that by nature, occupational therapy practitioners are creative. To be an effective occupational therapy practitioner, one practices FORTE on a daily basis, whether in the clinic, in the classroom as an instructor, in the administration as a department manager or in the lab as a researcher. Occupational therapy practitioners are generally flexible in working with others as we create the treatment plans or guide others in setting their personal goals. We exhibit open-mindedness when we listen to our staff, students, patients, the patient's family and others in considering all options. We often combine risk-taking with our tolerance for ambiguity as we look to the future and create goals that reflect the context in which we are working. What we do on a daily basis necessitates that we demonstrate empathy. We mindfully shift our point of view to that of the staff, students, client, caregiver and others involved with a particular situation. We work in a collaborative effort with our clients, students and subordinates to create meaningful and successful futures that overcome challenges of those individuals to whom we are responsible.

However, what I also wanted to include in the talk was an assessment of the ways in which the terrorists exemplified (from a creative thinker's point of view) a FORTE for creativity. To accomplish what they did (albeit as evil an act as it was); the terrorists had to be *flexible* as a group and as individuals. Although they had different values and belief systems than we have in America, did they not exhibit flexibility to fit into our society without, for the most part, making them obvious and

suspicious? We can only wonder how they might have exhibited flexibility as to where, how, and when they would carry out their act of terrorism had there been an airline flight delay due to equipment problems
or unfavorable weather conditions. On the other hand, we can only
wonder whether there *were* flight delays on the "original" day of the
"plan" and September 11 was in fact the alternate date! One thing that
does seem apparent; there appeared to be no flexibility in what they
chose to be their "targets."

Were not the terrorists demonstrating their ability to be *open-minded*
and blindly trust their leaders when they accepted an assignment without knowing the exact circumstances in which they would be acting? As
was reported in the news media regarding those 19 men, who turned the
airplanes into weapons against us on September 11, the hijackers to-be
were recruited for a mission without knowing the magnitude or scope of
their mission.

The ultimate challenge that the hijackers faced was that once the mission began, there was no turning back. Their demonstration of being a
risk taker was evident. If the mission was accomplished, death was a
certainty. (From our Western way of thinking, death is not a welcome
opportunity; from those who believe in being rewarded in the afterlife,
the prospect of dying has a very different interpretation). If the hijackers
were captured, they potentially faced spending the rest of their lives in
an American prison. If they did not accomplish the mission, there is a
high probability that they would die at the hands of their fellow terrorists.

Each terrorist took numerous risks of getting caught by United States
authorities on the way to their respective airports. They risked being
caught by immigration upon entering the United States. They risked being questioned by the property owners when they rented apartments or
by rental agents when they rented vehicles in the United States. Were
not the terrorists taking a risk of being questioned by authorities when
they used cash to purchase one-way tickets for their respective flights?
There were risks communicating with members of their terrorist cell in
efforts to coordinate the timing of the attacks. And once they took the
risk of clearing the gates on their way to entering each of the respective
airplanes, they risked that the passengers on four different flights would
not thwart their actions.

Creative thinking is a tool for managing change. The changes that
came about to the world following September 11, 2001–whether they
are airport or train security for travel or our personal shifts in the choices
we make whether to engage in social events that involve crowds or

working in a tall building—were creative. The terrorist acts on America were creative. They manifested a change that we are only beginning to comprehend. However, these thoughts needed to be left unspoken so soon after the events.

Was not their act to blindly accept this assignment a demonstration of having a *tolerance for ambiguity*? The hijackers had no way of knowing that they were on a suicide-mission-in-training. They were sent to flight school to learn to fly, without concern for taking off or landing the plane (as reported later by one flight school instructor where one of the hijackers of September 11 trained). Were they told by their leaders that they did not need to learn to take off and land a plane and their blind trust of their superiors was enough not to question them? Or were they in fact aware that they might at some time in the future commandier a suicide flight, just not know exactly which one? Whatever the case, their actions of September 11 demonstrated their tolerance for ambiguity.

And in what way did the hijackers demonstrate *empathy*—an important attribute of the creative thinker. They certainly did not exhibit empathy for the American people. On the other hand, if you shift your point of view to that of the terrorists, might not their horrific acts be framed as "empathy" for those people in their homeland? They represented people who hate everything, which the United States of America represents. The terrorists were willing to risk their own lives, the ultimate sacrifice (from our perspective) to cause great harm to what they perceived to be a financial symbol of the United States' wealth, the World Trade towers, and our military strength, the Pentagon.

In the keynote, I wanted to express thoughts on the security aspects of 9/11. The thoughts that follow were formulated, yet relating them to the attendees was a personal risk I was not ready to take. For the Ohio presentation, I created a five-minute video animation to introduce the concept of thinking-out-of-the-box. Creative thinkers think out-of-the-box and essentially think differently than others. The more I thought about the attacks and specifically how our security was compromised on September 11, I was struck by the fact that what the terrorists did was a very out-of-the-box act. "You don't know what you don't know," a quote I once heard from a corporate presenter, crept into my consciousness. The actions of the terrorists were out of OUR box or way of thinking.

There were all sorts of security opportunities that American authorities overlooked simply because the actions of the terrorists was a clear example of "out-of-the-box thinking" with regard to American culture. Similar to the other thoughts that remained unspoken, the analogy of the terrorist attack to out-of-the-box thinking would just as well have been inappropriate so close to the event. Until September 11, the terrorists' actions were inconceivable to us. The terrorists were clearly operating out of a different paradigm or "box" from ours. They had a way of thinking that permitted them to KMF, keep moving forward. They apparently moved along the route to accomplishing their mission without triggering suspicion by their personal demeanor or actions.

As for the yellow buttons proclaiming, "I am a human becoming," I believe that we have just begun to experience the ways in which this statement is taking on a life of its own. The statement on the yellow buttons is even more true to our way of living than the day that they were distributed to the participants at the November 2001 keynote. More so today than in the months immediately following the attacks on America, we are becoming a less-trusting-of-our-fellow-person society. We are learning to be hyper vigilant when in crowds. Some of us are rethinking our travel plans and whether we are ready to board an airplane with the assurance that we will arrive safely at our destination. We are becoming accustomed to periodic announcements by governmental officials that we are under a "nonspecific terrorist alert." Yet, the announcements encourage us that we should go on with our normally planned activities! We are changing and "becoming" in the course of everything that we do.

Perhaps some day, when adjusted to the "New World" that began after the attacks on America September 11, 2001, the context of an audience will support the thoughts expressed above. Until that time, I will continue to be astounded at the impact that the terrorists' creative thinking had on the world. In addition, I hope that those who serve to protect and guard our nation's safety develop their FORTE for creative thinking. Today more than ever before, we need to move "out of our box" as we learn to understand others with different values that motivate actions that are unacceptable for the good and well-being of humanity.

REFERENCES

Caine, R. & Caine, G. (1994). *Making connections: Teaching and the human brain.* New York: Addison-Wesley.

Lewin, J. & Reed, C. (1998). *Creative problem solving in occupational therapy.* Philadelphia, PA: Lippincott Williams & Wilkins.

Smith, R. (1997). *The 7 levels of change.* Arlington, TX: The Summit Publishing Group.

Index

BOOK ORDER FORM!

Order a copy of this book with this form or online at:
http://www.haworthpress.com/store/product.asp?sku=5690

Healing 9/11

Creative Programming by Occupational Therapists

_____ in softbound at $19.95 ISBN-13: 978-0-7890-2363-6 / ISBN-10: 0-7890-2363-6.
_____ in hardbound at $34.95 ISBN-13: 978-0-7890-2362-9 / ISBN-10: 0-7890-2362-8.

COST OF BOOKS _____

POSTAGE & HANDLING _____
US: $4.00 for first book & $1.50
for each additional book
Outside US: $5.00 for first book
& $2.00 for each additional book.

SUBTOTAL _____
In Canada: add 7% GST. _____

STATE TAX _____
CA, IL, IN, MN, NJ, NY, OH, PA & SD residents
please add appropriate local sales tax.

FINAL TOTAL _____
If paying in Canadian funds, convert
using the current exchange rate,
UNESCO coupons welcome.

❑**BILL ME LATER:**
Bill-me option is good on US/Canada/
Mexico orders only; not good to jobbers,
wholesalers, or subscription agencies.

❑**Signature** _____

❑**Payment Enclosed: $** _____

❑ **PLEASE CHARGE TO MY CREDIT CARD:**
❑Visa ❑MasterCard ❑AmEx ❑Discover
❑Diner's Club ❑Eurocard ❑ JCB

Account # _____

Exp Date _____

Signature _____
(Prices in US dollars and subject to change without notice.)

PLEASE PRINT ALL INFORMATION OR ATTACH YOUR BUSINESS CARD

Name	
Address	
City	State/Province Zip/Postal Code
Country	
Tel	Fax
E-Mail	

May we use your e-mail address for confirmations and other types of information? ❑Yes ❑No We appreciate receiving
your e-mail address. Haworth would like to e-mail special discount offers to you, as a preferred customer.
We will never share, rent, or exchange your e-mail address. We regard such actions as an invasion of your privacy.

Order from your **local bookstore** or directly from
The Haworth Press, Inc. 10 Alice Street, Binghamton, New York 13904-1580 • USA
Call our toll-free number (1-800-429-6784) / Outside US/Canada: (607) 722-5857
Fax: 1-800-895-0582 / Outside US/Canada: (607) 771-0012
E-mail your order to us: orders@haworthpress.com

For orders outside US and Canada, you may wish to order through your local
sales representative, distributor, or bookseller.
For information, see http://haworthpress.com/distributors

(Discounts are available for individual orders in US and Canada only, not booksellers/distributors.)

Please photocopy this form for your personal use.
www.HaworthPress.com

BOF05